The New Science Of Psychiatrical Engineering

Psychiatry and Schizophrenia Based On Physics

By Jamil Kazoun
(Jamil Talaat Malak Sukkarieh Kazoun)

Version 1
Copyright 2018. All rights reserved.

Forward

Before humans knew of the existence of bacteria few years ago, did bacteria not exist? Then after they discovered them, they realized they are the cause of much disease. Then after, discovered some cures for them. Same for viruses, more recently. Same for fungus. All were completely unknown or like fiction before their discovery under the microscope. Now, you will learn that there are still other undiscovered creatures, called spirits. Some are much smaller, and some of them cause diseases, especially psychiatric diseases, and most specifically, cause schizophrenia.

Your knowledge regarding spirits as most professionals and layman is likely to be nearly non-existent beyond what is known from the religious realm. No science or very little hints of it provides this knowledge. So how do I begin this monumental task of educating on such a new and considerably unknown subject, a subject that is also looked at by many as the domain of fiction, speculation, religion, and suspicion. And how do I set the ground so that scientists can look at the subject in a scientific manner, and especially to look at it as an engineering subject, to be tackled in a most rigorous scientific way based on physics? I think the task is very difficult since the hurdles are many, but my hope is that you will keep your mind open until the argument is completely presented before you rush to judgment. It is an extremely new subject, and you have to be patient to read the entire argument before you close the door on this. I will repeat it several times because it is so important to keeping your mind open: In history, no bacteria was known, then it became known, then associated with disease, then precise medicine is discovered to kill it. We are going thru the same process now for viruses, and fungus. All relatively new to medicine and science. Scientists and laymen also believed for thousands of years, that the sun revolved around the earth, but the exact opposite was true! Same for today's psychiatry, its solutions are exactly the opposite of what is the true cause of the problems. Schizophrenia for example for the most part is not a chemical or neurological imbalance, or such, but is a spirit related imbalance and problem. You are about to possibly throw away most if not all of your understanding of the subject, so prepare to listen with an open mind, for your own sake, and for the sake of patients. Read thru, and read several times if you must. It is this important and it is this new!

I will need to speak about new beings, creatures completely unknown to scientists and laymen, about their physical properties, locations, and touch on religion as a bit of connecting point, because religion has been almost the only area that spoke of these beings. Even religions spoke so little and so vaguely and so uselessly for scientists about the subject, but one thing religions did, and almost all universally implied, that they exist, by speaking of them. Scientists and engineers did not take the logical step of asking, "if" and "only if" they exist, and I being a scientist and possibly a believer in some of these religions, I owe it to myself to ask the logical question: "If" they exist, and I am not sure, where do they exist at? What is their location? And what is their form? Because if they exist, they must have a location, and a form! But scientists have been blinded from exploring this possibility, and for now, in this introduction, we will leave this as a possibility about "If they exist", and later in the book move to know that "They most certainly do exist! And we will understand the consequences and fantastic opportunities in treating patients, understanding our world, and learn how to develop new highly advanced technologies that will take medicine and science way beyond today's technology."

A creature usually has a form, needs energy source to survive or move, sometimes a fixed location as a home, etc. That is never addressed usually by religion, beyond merely using the term they are in "heaven or heavens", "Celestial world", "spirit world", etc. , as their location, and nothing about their physical body, and how they can move, function and interact with humans. I will look at all this from a strictly physics perspective not a metaphysical perspective. I will want laboratory tools and microscopes as investigation tools, not the speculation and guessing of today's psychiatry. These maybe sharp words for some in the field, but do not get offended at the risk of staying ignorant, just like other scientists before thought the earth is flat, the sun revolves around the earth, and had no knowledge that there exists such tiny creatures as bacteria and viruses, etc. They were wrong, and held to their wrong believes so strongly!

While humans inhabit a physical piece of land, bacteria inhabits a human. And a spirit can inhabit a bacteria or a human or space. So the heavens, or celestial world, or the spirit world, can be in part a human body. Much is done from these heavens, unknowingly. And some of these spirits are intelligent and some incredibly intelligent, just as some are not. That is the reality, not what some unknowing person dreams or imagines it to be. I need to deal with the religion subject and other subjects as much as needed for some understanding, touched upon for foundational background even if done once at the foundation of a new science. But the focus and the ONLY method that will be sought, is physics as the tool and the logic to guide and investigate. So let us start.

I hope many will benefit from this book.
Jamil Kazoun

March 21, 2018

This book is mostly a compilation from my other work. The order of chapters is, for the most part, not coherent. Not much attention is given to composition or other editorial and grammatical elements. There is only the need to publish the book fast to make it available to readers. My situation is extremely difficult health wise, and I am barely able to dedicate my energy and focus as I wish. I can hardly work to type at the computer or manage my daily chores. My problems are compounded by lack of resources available to me so I cannot get the needed help in my life, or work on the book in a leisurely fashion, for composition, editing, and completeness. While I cannot hand you the whole tree, the fruits you will get should be enough as a great starting point.

Forgive my mistakes, of disorganization of chapters or paragraphs or grammatical or spelling errors if any. That is not important and is trivial in such a new work, and under the severe personal health struggle from spirits that I face to be able to get the books out. Keep your mind focused on the important elements that make the big picture and the facts. This book talks about spirits, a life form you likely know absolutely nothing about, and a world you have not seen so far - the world of the spirits. This book may be the first of its kind.

The spirit world is practically unknown to most. Its secrets usually unavailable or inaccessible to us. This book offers a window and a big door into this world, giving details not easily found, so that doctors, scientists and engineers can look, understand, and create needed tools and solutions for patients. For those suffering from this spirit world: the people who were or are labeled schizophrenics, those who hear voices in their head, those who see internally imposed images or spirits that others cannot see, or those who feel strange sensations in or on their body; this book has much to explain so that they can understand their situation or to help professionals understand their situation, to help finding solutions to their problem.

Even though at first it may seem strange and not like the proper place for this book to talk about advanced technology, I do so as an absolute and necessary byproduct of the spirits subject, as creatures that are technologically advanced, and delve into the related subject of future computers and robots built based on advanced non-solid state electromagnetic structures, similar to some types of spirits, and how these robots can travel to the planets in minutes, even seconds, instead of years, go inside human bodies to explore, see, and fix problems, without human skin being cut open, and how to communicate with them, externally or internally, and how to go underwater or under earth and thru hard structures without difficulties. This is incidental because in the hunt for spirits that torture schizophrenics, people who are said to have schizophrenia, and are suffering from spirits, it is important to understand beings made completely from electromagnetic fields and these beings' capabilities.

Jamil

Creating the Center For Psychiatrical Engineering

Psychiatry in its current status is an art form full of misunderstanding of the factors underlying major psychiatric problems such as schizophrenia. My goal is to transform psychiatry into an engineering science based on physics. My central assertion is that the problem of so-called schizophrenia is caused by spirits, living entities that are part of human life, and solving the problem of schizophrenia would be through attacking or dealing with those spirits. Humans lived a long time with bacteria, maybe not knowing they exist and they populate the body (skin, mouth, intestines, etc.), and maybe for thousands of years, were helpless against bacterial diseases. They neither knew of bacteria nor that the bacteria was causing the problem. It was not until relatively recently that they learned about bacteria and that many are actually in the body and part of the normal function. And it was not until very recently after discovering bacteria that anti-bacterial medicine was discovered and developed. Similarly for viruses, being unknown, then after become known, and now in the process of developing antiviral medication. Our assertion is that spirits, entities that some are much smaller than viruses also populate human beings and maybe part of the normal function, and just like bacteria, when they are bad, they can cause illness such as schizophrenia. We have to discover them, their locations, and create anti spirit solutions. For thousands of years most also believed the earth was flat, and that "the sun revolved around the earth", and the scientist that told them it was the opposite "the earth revolved around the sun", was imprisoned, and later proven correct. You will come to see that this is the case also here.

We aim to lay the foundation needed to achieve this goal by:
Providing new information about the real causes of psychiatric disorders, and specifically, we will be focused on what is called "schizophrenia" as a difficult problem for those suffering from it.
Provide lists of relevant tools and equipment to investigate researchers' hypotheses.
List the needed research areas to comprehensively cover the spectrum of possibilities in the search for solutions.
Be a platform for information on latest ongoing research, and the needed research areas that should be worked on.
Be a place that facilitates finding needed talent and resources
Be a place that promotes research into this problem, in order to find a solution to it.

Definition of Psychiatrical Engineering: Psychiatry based on physics. The underlying principal is "when there is a sound heard, there is a source for it. Finding the location of the source generating the sound is the beginning for finding a solution". Similarly for images and sensations. I created the new term and field.

About me

It is not known by the public in general how much a person who has so-called schizophrenia suffers. The suffering can be non-stop and for every waking minute of their day. And sometimes, even suffering while asleep from nightmares, unpleasant dreams, or sleep paralysis or spirit attacks. There is also the stigma by some cultures about such mysterious problems, and fears of being labeled as crazy, etc. Factors that prevents some sufferers from talking about their problem at all, or openly, especially publically. In severe cases, people, even when looking very healthy physically, like myself, sometimes may become practically completely disabled, unable to focus on work or tasks, or earn a living, or take care of themselves or others. After knowing this, it is hard not to be motivated to help, and do something about this problem if possible. This book and center are a result of this. I thank the many that helped survive and deal with this experience, of humans and spirits, and I hope you can take some satisfaction from the results. I hope these results will not be corrupted or diluted in the future, by the same evil spirits that fought me to prevent these revelations.

Action Plans

The center is built on the believe that

the proper central hypothesis to propose and investigate, that is scientific, and will lead to a solution to the problem of schizophrenia, is this:

Fact:

"Whenever there is a sound (or image or sensation) heard (seen, felt), there is a source generating the sound, and there is a location for this source."

Questions to answer:

1. Where is the location of this sound source?

2. How is the sound being generated?

AND

3. What is the location of the area hearing the sound?

Answering these most basic questions, are the foundation of laying the grounds for scientific research into this problem,

and the first step in finding a solution. When we know, we can investigate these locations, and target them as needed.

Example 1: Sound Waves

- Firecracker is burned somewhere unknown. Sound waves are generated → Technical Equipment 1 kilometer away Hears the sound, and determines exact location of the sound.

  Firecrackers are located. People lighting the firecrackers are located, and catched.

Example 2: Electromagnetic Waves

- Cell phone is stolen and used somewhere unknown. Electromagnetic waves are generated → Technical Equipment hundreds of kilometers away Detect the waves, and determines exact location of the wave source.

  Phone is located. People using the phone are located, and catched.

Helping Patients .... *Transforming Psychiatry Into a Science*

Example 3:

Sound is heard inside a patient's mind

Internal firecracker sound is heard inside patient's head.

Sound waves
or
electromagnetics waves
or
chemical messenger molecules are generated to carry the wave from unknown source to unknown destination (internal ear of patient) Using an unknown medium or pathway for the transmission

→

Technical Equipment to detect sound location cannot be placed inside the patient's internal ear to hear the sound.

And we do not know the exact spot for the internal ear if we could insert the equipment or an electric probe, or non-invasive probe

Therefore, the sound source cannot be located.

How do we solve this problem?

What are available options?

Do we take a completely different approach than this traditional method of sound location?

If we can solve this problem, we would have solved the first and big part of the puzzle. The second part then becomes catching the source generating the sound from this spot. These creatures are extremely tiny. But the task should be achievable.
Our problem is solved. The patient can be helped by destroying the source, convincing it not to harrass the patient, other options available.

Our Research and Grants

Research Areas and Grants

1. Location identification of sound origin: identify available tools for identifying the source of a sound. Making a list of such equipment, Manufacturer, cost, equipment specifications , and identifying the relevant factors in such a search (wave type such as pressure sound wave, etc. frequency, frequency type, etc.) To help researchers in the field find needed tool to investigate hypotheses.

2. Transmission of sound to the ear, direct and indirect, external thru air , audible and inaudible such as thru ultrasounds, x-ray or MRI. Identifying possible ways for such transmissions and the factors involved in transmission such as the effect of the medium in the ear and around it, and relevant pathways leading to it such as nerve pathways, blood pathways and vein membranes, etc. Pain nerve pathways, endocrine pathways, etc, completely identifying all know system that connect to the ear.

3. Organizing and summarizing all important research findings so far related to ability to generate in-ear sounds and words to a person using inaudible frequency range equipment. And relevant ear and brain regions, and structures. This list will be used by researchers to formulate hypotheses and test the hypotheses.

4. Identifying available equipment that scan wide frequency ranges for programmable characteristics, such as used by science centers scanning for intelligent-communication signals in outer space. How to possibly modify such equipment or create new equipment able to scan for sound related activities in the ear, it's surrounding areas, external or internal, pathways to it, and relevant brain regions, and central nerve system relevant factors. This list gives researches a starting point to identify, collaborate, purchase or create needed equipment with the required specifications to allow the to conduct their research.

5. Use of sound frequencies, audible or inaudible to suppress internal sounds heard by patients. From heavy duty industrial equipment suitable for clinics, to over the counter cell phone applications available for anyone such as "ToneGenerator" that can create frequencies in range of 1hz to 20khz in different waveforms and specifications, and can repeatedly sweep thru the frequencies". If effective, why? What the location of the ear part, brain, or nerves effected? Etc. This to help patients suppress unwanted internally generated sounds, and to look at the problem of identifying the internal generated sound sources and areas from a different angle.

6. Use of magnets frequencies, or magnetic or electric fields to suppress internal sounds heard by patients. From heavy duty industrial equipment suitable for clinics, to over the counter magnet balls available for anyone in different sizes and shapes, to put in

proximity of a patient's ear or other body parts to test for any effect. If effective, why? What is the location involved, other factors, etc. If patient internally generated sounds have an electric or magnetic component in this process, magnetic or electric fields disturbing this process may give some clues in the search for the source of these sounds and method of transmission. This help patients suppress unwanted internally generated sounds, and to look at the problem of identifying the internal generated sound sources and areas from a different angle.

10. For those interested in generating electromagnetic wave structures for robots, it maybe worth noting that two magnets, one round and one elliptical touching each other, are being held together by magnetic force. If a slight force is placed in the edge of the elliptical magnet, it will rotate like the blade of an airplane propeller, while still attached by magnetic force. This gives a very primitiveness idea about how two structures can be attached to each other magnetically. Can you translate this into the electromagnetic field area to join structures? Play with different shapes and structures, and identify analogies and relevant mathematics involved to create general hypotheses for other researches more skilled in other areas to get involved, create hypotheses, and test them, to help create the founding blocks in mathematics, and physics to create these new robotic and computer machines. An electric current or signal creates a magnetic field and a magnetic field can create electric

Signal. A transformer can transmit power wirelessly between two coils? I do not know where to start, but anything, anything, that may prompt an idea in another scientist in St mind may be useful to put down as we randomly or intently search to find and create needed ideas and tools to kick start this process.

11. Looking for electromagnetic receptors. Receptors that expect the transmitter to be extremely near at the cell level, and other receptors that are sensitive to transmissions from very far distances. Receivers at micro cell level and molecular size levels. And larger ones in the base of the spine and bellow it. Waves that cover the entire spine or body, and with multiple large waves that together converge on one target tiny spot (as in Fourier wave transforms that target a discrete space) etc. The ways are many. Grants for the same, but for receptors for light (instead of sound), as a communication reception mechanism. Some spirits I saw used light communication.

Spirits, robotics, and schizophrenia

Sometimes when you are trying to get to a specific place and you cannot get there, you have to create new tools to reach that location. So when some human beings decided to go to the moon they did not have the tools to get there. Neither horses nor cars nor trains nor ships could get them there. They had to invent space rockets and space shuttles and this took them into outer space and planets, and specifically to the moon, and they landed there.
Similarly I think people did not know about bacteria and viruses until only few hundred years ago, and they had no understanding of these things and have never seen them. Later on with the discovery of microscopes and other new tools such as x-ray machines and MRI etc. they could see these beings and also they could develop antibiotics or additional tools to understand and to control them.

This shows the importance of new inventions that are not available technologically now to reach a new destination.
Similarly if we want to understand the spirit world as it relates to schizophrenia, in our assertion that spirits are the main component of that problem, then we need to understand spirits' construction or function, and how they move and interact. From this perspective it's very important to make a big jump from psychiatry and schizophrenia into the spirit world and from there into the field of electromagnetic robotics, in order to see and understand spirits. Towards that goal, we need to start by understanding the not yet invented field of electromagnetic robotics. When we understand electromagnetic robotics then we can take the next step to start the hunt for these spirits and their location in a scientific manner.
When you look at your skin with your naked eye do you see any of the millions of bacteria on it? When you look at your mouth and the saliva in it, or if you spit that saliva outside, do you see any of the millions of bacteria in it? Similarly for the bacteria in your intestines, etc. Millions and millions of them, on you, or in you, and you do not see them or feel them.
Same for viruses, or fungus, etc.

Also, the millions and millions of electromagnetic waves touching you or going inside your body every moment. Do you see them? Do you feel them? But if you placed a radio next to you, then you can detect some of them, in some frequency ranges, and listen to what they are carrying in sound information, so-to-speak. So you listen to the radio. But the radio signal is electromagnetic, and is near you, and is also touching your skin and body, and is also going inside your body, and part of it is going thru your body. So millions of electromagnetic waves carrying sound are constantly touching your body and going inside it. Similarly for tv waves, and here, millions of electromagnetic waves are touching your body and going inside it. These are electromagnetic waves carrying sound and images and moving images touch your body and go inside it. You may say, Wow! Interesting! I am starting to get a sense that I will have a new understand coming, and starting to see a pattern that will help me reach this understanding.

So let us move on. Remember or do you know that maybe only fifty years ago, a solid-state transistor was the size of your finger, and now it is so small, you cannot see it with the naked eye, and millions of it can fit on your finger? That is what a modern computer chip is made from. Before, the transistor was made as a glass tube, and now it is made as a silicon-based structure that is extremely small, invisible to the naked eye. Now, can you imagine a transistor made from electromagnetic material? From electromagnetic waves? Just like we make radio and TV signals from electromagnetic wave material? If yes, then great. Now we have a structure that can move in space, carry information AND PROCESS information! It is invisible, super-fast in travel, will enter your body, and can touch your skin, and the skin of all the people in your city, or your country, and earth if need be and the signal is strong enough. So what is a computer made on a single silicon chip? Many transistors linked together to store and process information. Well, instead of a single electromagnetic transistor let us talk about a single electromagnetic wave-material computer. Not a big jump in imagining or technological invention maybe. The problem with a silicon transistor or a silicon computer chip is that it cannot move by itself. It needs a human being to carry it from the store to the house, for example. But an electromagnetic computer can be transported easy, without human intervention. The store will broadcast it to your home , just like a radio station or TV station broadcast the signal to your home. But such a transmission is primitive, one way and simple, from sender to receivers.

We need to go one more step for the interesting stuff. Few years ago I had a robot in my home that cleans the floor by itself with no guidance from me. It moves around the room cleaning the floor. Very inexpensive. Robots are very common now in industrial applications and some are available for personal use. A robot is simply a computer that has mechanical parts that can move, such as arms, legs, wheels, propulsion engines, eyes, ears, touch sensors, sonars, etc. If we learn to create mechanical parts made from electromagnetic material, then creating a robot made entirely from electromagnetic material becomes possible.

This robot by being made from electromagnetic material will have these qualities:
Super lightweight with its weight being almost zero
Super-fast in moving. Can move anywhere on earth in a fraction of a second, and to outer space and planets in seconds or minutes.
Can touch the bodies of one human being, or all persons in a city or a country or earth.
Can go inside the human body to see or do something inside it (medical or otherwise) or simply to pass through it or through barriers etc.
Can go into deep oceans, underneath the earth, to investigate or look at things. Same for going to the moon or other places
The same robot can be extremely small in size and then in an instant change its shape to become extremely large just like a radio or tv signal generated small to instantly enlarge to cover thousands of square or cubic kilometers in size.
Its shape is extremely flexible and can morph to any shape needed near instantly. So are its extremities.
Such a robot becomes like the spirits I am acquainted with, in terms of form and functionality.
Spirits are real! All around us in unbelievable numbers, forms, shapes, intelligence, and other qualities. They are part of us, related to us, and some maybe in most personal and intimate ways. Some are very good, some very evil, and some indifferent, and many

nearly robot-like in function. With this said, I will go no further to remain focused on the problem at hand, which is, finding a solution, a permanent one, to those suffering schizophrenia, hearing voices, etc.

All this background and more tools will be needed just to address this problem at its roots. Just like going to the moon and a seeing a bacteria or virus required inventing and manufacturing new very sophisticated tools, this is the same case here. But the job is doable, and can be achieved possibly in very short time. It is irrelevant the time frame as this must be done, for patients with tremendous suffering, let alone the incredible technological advances and economic riches that will come from such technology and will drive this field when understood. Also, this field has other very deep ramifications about us as human beings.

Definition of Electromagnetic (EM) Computers: Computers made entirely from non solid state electromagnetic wave parts. They have no electronic or optical or solid state parts, etc. . This is a new term I created for a new field in computer design and manufacturing that I thought of.

Definition of Electromagnetic Robots: EM computers that can move controllably in space and have sensors and/or moving parts and forms. This is a new term I created for a new field in robotics design and manufacturing that I thought of. More details can be found in my books.

Fears and Apprehension From a New Field and Technology

The fears government and people may have when brain control or transmission tools become widely available:

What if your neighbor decided to use his new over the counter tool to transmit evil speech to you, unwanted and without permission? What if he decided to send you a fear impulse in one second or sex arousal impulse. How do you deal with all this?

I do not want to. I will leave this subject to others. What is important is to not let fear hold us back, and hold back science. We should create all these tools, and during or after, as problems arise, create solutions to the new problems. A knife is used every day by many to eat. That someone may choose to use it to hurt someone else is not a reason not to make knives and use them widely. Do not inhibit the full fledge development of this new field because of fear. Just as the answer in a democracy for bad speech is more speech, not less, this is also the case. There are cost benefit analysis to many areas, and we should err on the side of freedom and knowledge, and find tools to deal with arising issues.

Military and Classified research

Because extremely important research is done in a classified (secret) manner in the area of brain activity, it is important to write a note about this.

A message to non lethal military weapon researchers and companies involved in classified research and tools production:

It is well established that voice (auditory) transmission from equipment (at microwave or other frequency levels) directly to a person's inner ear is possible. For military use, these researchers understand that an enemy soldier can be paralyzed by such transmissions. (https://www.wired.com/2008/02/report-nonletha/   a newly declassified Pentagon report, Bioeffects of Selected Non-Lethal Weapons, obtained by a private citizen under the Freedom of Information Act, provides some fascinating tidbits on a variety of exotic weapons ideas. Among those discussed are weapons that could disrupt the brain) and (http://transmissionsmedia.com/the-voice-of-god-nonlethal-weapons-could-target-brain-mimic-schizophrenia/   basis to this technology? Well, Holosonic Research Labs and American Technology Corporation both have versions of directed sound, which can allow a single person to hear a message that others around don't hear. DARPA appears to be working on its own sonic projector. Intriguingly, Strategy Page reports that troops are using the Long Range Acoustic Device as a modified Voice of God weapon:) and (http://www.newworldwar.org/microwavehearing.htm   July of 2008 New Scientist announced that Sierra Nevada Corporation planned to build a microwave gun able to project beams of sounds directly into people's heads)

The constant voices these soldiers would hear and types of words and their volume can paralyze them or greatly distract their focus to make them unable to function properly or at peak performance. Also additional transmissions can effect their physical body and sensations to further disable the soldier. This can be done. It is important for you to understand that a person suffering Schizophrenia faces the "exact" problem!!!!! He is being harassed, made to loose focus, by voices he hears (or things he sees or sensations he feels). You as classified military weapon researchers know how to create the problem. Now I ask you to please help create the solution. At the simplest and most expediate level, the solution can be to use the same machine that can create the problem to "suppress" the existing ongoing unwanted voices in a patient's head. The same tool used to transmit frequencies to transmit sound can be use to do the opposite, to suppress or cover the other sounds, or send pleasing sounds that are stronger than the unwanted sounds. There are many options to help these people whose sufferings you can or cannot imagine. Help these people, these patients!!!!

Making your research and tools completely open to civilians is far more important to serve people, your country, and possibly your financial success, or your conscious. You can still make these as weapons for the military and police. A country's military can loose some advantages making these civilian tools, but this civilian gain far out-ways the military benefits which ultimately is supposed to serve civilians! A country is not always at war, but is mostly always at peace (in civilian status) and its civilians need these tools to be used every day to comfort them, more than the few days of war that may or may not happen some day, and these tools may or may not be put to use.

Put your research and tools to use now and everyday, to help your own civilian citizens, not keep them in secret to be used on rare occasions and in few incidents. There may be little financial, or moral logic in such actions. There may be military logic to your actions or motivation, but no civil logic or motivation. Please think about this proposition thoroughly and move swiftly to implement it. Millions of people, patients, need help and you can do so greatly! Let alone the other benefits that come from civilians being aware of all that is possible and civilians being in control of it. If you are a military person in charge of such research, you should understand the importance of this underlying principal in an open, transparent, healthy, democratic society. The transfer of this military technology and knowledge should be done swiftly to civilian companies and researchers for a healthier people, and economy. As a company, sell your equipment to many hospitals, doctors, and countries. Military equipment does not need to pass civilian agencies safety standards, and this can complicate things, but the financial rewards should be commensurate or made to be. Knowing that you will be helping millions of people whose lives are a living hell may also give you some satisfaction.

Motivations to researchers, entrepreneurs, visionaries:

It has been well known by science and medicine for many years that a physical probe inserted in the brain at the appropriate location can make a person feel or hear or see things. Alternatively, this probe can be used to make you hear good things or stop bad voices, and make you feel relaxed and happy as counter measure to feeling anxiety and fear or pain. 1. Sensations (fear, happiness, relaxation,etc), and remembrances (the smell of an apple, the sound of a river they knew, the face of a relative, etc..), and to hear words. To hear complete sentences may require transmitting not just one electric pulse, but a train of pulses, with specific time spread, shape, energy level, encoding etc. But it can be done. So almost any direct sensory or mental reception can be directly simulated, and this should be logical and expected. The problem is not scientists doing this to solve human problems, but evil spirits doing it for bad purposes, such as control a human or abuse them. Their simulation can be more complicated, because it can be indirect, by transmission of electromagnetic energy, directly to the area, or to the nerves that will stimulate the area. So instead of sending a pulse to the base of the brain, they can do this at any area along the spine that connect to the base of the brain.

Do the same with an external noninvasive probe. Use an electromagnetic signal directed at the correct area. We can solve untold problems for patients this way. And can do much more in other areas as well. A kidney stone needed invasive surgery to get to it in the past to remove it, now this can be done by waves from the outside, breaking the stone and pissing it out, by sound waves, or other waves. Find solutions! If it is a function or sensation for a human, than it likely has a location in the brain (or spine etc.), And has representation and possibly encoding. Find the location, discover the representation, and break the encoding if any. Then use this to solve problems. And let us move on with medicine (and our view of our-self, and life itself).

Schizophrenia and Stigma: effects on research

Stigma is a major hurdle that must be overcome in patients for them to be able gain ability to seek help, and for them to help researchers, and to help educate the public. Evil spirits know and use stigma against patients, to keep them isolated, suffering in secret. Seeking openness strengthens patients and gives them the chance to recover and have a somewhat normal life. Without this, their chance of healing may be lower, and take longer, suffering more. Stigma should be overcome, and patients should be taught the importance of being open and relaxed about discussing their condition.

Stigma has important effect on research, in not allowing researchers to know all interesting cases that can be learned from. Also, stigma may prevent a patient from openly sharing completely the details of his problem, thus, prevent a full understand of the problem and finding a solution. Patients such as these maybe a great asset to researchers because they are the one that have active spirits, and when these spirits are active, they can be listened to talking or doing other things, and hopefully located. These patients with ongoing severe problems can be the best key to solving this puzzle.

Research efforts are by others just beginning

Here is one study to identify the problem. But typically, they have no idea what the problem is:

Tuning in to the Voices: A Multisite fMRI (Functional MRI) Study of Auditory Hallucinations
https://www.ncbi.nlm.nih.gov/pmc/articles/PMC2643968/

http://www.psychiatricalengineering.org/research-by-others

Famous People With Schizophrenia

Brian Wilson	Co-founder of the Beach Boys music band	Hears voices. Torture him.	Spoke publicly about his problem. He SUFFERED for a long time. He still was able to compose beautiful music, but said if the suffering was worth it to compose beautiful music, he said "no"!!!!!! Stay away from this world! This is not for games or experimentation!!!! https://youtu.be/OLdjjXDtA8g
John Forbes Nash Jr.	Mathematician		John Forbes Nash Jr. (June 13, 1928 – May 23, 2015). Nobel Prize winner in economics. was an American mathematician who made fundamental contributions to] Nash's work has provided insight into the factors that govern chance and decision-making inside complex systems found in everyday life. https://youtu.be/Nxi7WZSLzUs
Abraham (, Beloved figure of Jews and Muslims)	Prophet? In Jewish Bible. Old Testament. Traditional Islam	Hearing voices	Hears a voice telling him to kill his innocent 12 year old boy. And goes to do it!!!!! He celebrated for this act with religious holidays
Buddha Sukyamooni	Buddha	Hearing voices by spirits he was seeing and communicating with	Even though he had access seemingly to much of the spirit world, and gave more than anyone I know knowledge about this world, he still during his development lacked knowledge (?) of what kind of food to eat. He became frail till spirits told him what to do .
Jesus	Prophet? (Lord?, god?) Or just a man or the son of man (a man)	Strange behavior pp people and family could not explain.	Some thought he had a devil in him, and his own family at times thought he was acting strange (crazy?). He and his cousin, while still in the womb, could hear and talk to each other.
Muhammad	Prophet of Islam religion	Hearing voices	In the cave, he heard a voice, supposedly of an angel, Gabriel?, And was told to read some writings even though he was illiterate in reading. At times, terrified from spirits, and one time, running to his wife sweating, asking her to cover him and comfort him
Moses	Prophet of the Jews	Hearing voices and seeing things	Hear voice telling him about the Ten Commandments and (sees a burning bush?)
John The Baptist	Jewish Religous figure	Seeing things in the spirit world	He saw a dove descend from heaven when he baptized Jesus
Vincent van Gogh	Famous painter	Hearing voices?	Cut off his ear. Was he trying to stop the unending and torturous voices by doing so? Try to imagine the suffering of some of these people!!!!!!!
Zelda Fitzgerald	Novelist and wife of F. Scott Fitzgerald, Zelda Fitzgerald		Source: https://m.ranker.com/list/famous-people-with-schizophrenia/celebrity-lists
Eduard Einstein	Son of Albert Einstein	Schizophrenia	https://m.ranker.com/list/famous-people-with-schizophrenia/celebrity-lists

Grants

Please specify the research topic/area from our list of research areas, or suggest a new area if needed, and apply. We aim to make the grant proposal very simple, in order to speed processing and issuing the grant. We hope grants can be approved and issued in a time frame of few days to few weeks at most. This is strictly for engineering type research, not social , psychological type research, or centrally-statistics-based research. We are looking for engineering-type research that includes equipment such as ultrasound, x ray, MRI, Ct Scan, electrode based, non-invasive based research that would allow us to locate the areas in which these sounds come from, and what are the inhabited organisms, material in that area. We suspect organisms/spirits extremely small in size, and possibly acting on micro single cell structures. We want physics-based engineering research in this pursuit. You also need access to psychiatric patients who suffered specifically from "hearing voices". The worse the patient's situation is, the better candidates they make. So having access to those who suffer from "constant commentary or hearing voices all the time they are awake" are best. So that when placed in a laboratory environment, there is good chance these nonstop taking voices will do so in the lab, and thus be subject to investigation. Therefore, since schizophrenic patients are required, and scientific tools and equipment are required, we highly encourage you to find scientists in other departments to collaborate with. If you are a psychiatrist find an an engineer or a physicist to work with. If you are an engineer or a physicist find a psychiatrist to work with.

For the grant application/proposal:
1. Be as specific as possible as to the area of research proposed
2. Give a summary statement about your research goal
3. A statement about how you plan to achieve your goals. Specify resources needed if any, equipment, etc.
4. Specify the time frame required to submit back to us your research findings, as a formal scientific research paper. The research findings need to be of a quality that they can be published in scientific journals.
5. Commitment to provide interim regularly timed updates about results and problems encountered so far. This will serve as part of this center being a place of interaction and allowing other researchers to provide you ongoing feedback about problems you may encounter, and to help with insights and other ways. We need the establish as much synergy as possible between researchers as this will greatly improve everyone's work. As part of the grant, if you desire, you will be given space on this website dedicated to your research with ability of others to comment on your work.
6. Include
    a. your name
    b. address
    c. email
    d. phone
    e. your institution
i. name
ii. address
iii. Department
    1. Name

	2.	phone
	3.	email
	4.	Department head name
	5.	department area of specialization
iv.	Supervisor if applicable and if different from above	
	1.	Name
	2.	Phone
	3.	Email
	4.	Title
	5.	Signature (an email from them can serve as signature)
	6.	if more than one supervisor is involved, please list also as above

To qualify you need to be: a PhD level researcher, or a professor. Exceptions will be made if there is good reason and it will benefit the research areas. Masters level candidates, and engineers, and physicists with BA level will be looked at if they have experience in areas being investigated and can provide useful information or tools for our purpose.

Is there a psychiatry department at your institution (University, hospital, clinic, institute, etc.)?

Include your relevant experience.

General awareness of the spirit world and its effect or interaction with humans

The western world today (such as the USA and Europe, considered as technologically highly advanced) are almost completely unaware of the existence of spirits and their interaction with humans. As seems to be the case in much of the rest of the world. There are few exceptions. Buddhist and Hindu related countries, such as Thailand, Laos, China, India seem to have relatively high level of knowledge, even if seemingly still very limited. Philippines was a big surprise to me in the widespread acceptance and awareness of Third Eye entity, and their understanding and practice of spirit transmigration by some. It should be noted that in Lebanon, my birth place and some neighbor countries, few did practice what is called "writing" where a person goes to a traditional spirit specialist person to write an ill-wish to a hated person, etc. to affect their life. Writings, that is planning ahead for the future seemed in my experience to be a natural and widespread practice of religion-related-spirits. That is, every religion has its own organized system, and writings are a part of it for some as a sort of plan for what they want to happen in the future of a person. In some South American countries such as Haiti, they are said to practice of voodoo.

Observations about Life

Meeting unseen loved ones or evil ones from distant and nearby spaces

The human body and those with the same properties, are not suitable for inter planet and interstellar travel. My experience shows that if we expect a UFO to be large, we are likely to be very disappointed. It would be better if we expect it and its occupants to be sub-nanometers in size and made from non-solid materials, perhaps made entirely from electromagnetic wave structures. Similar creatures seem already abundant on Earth.

The Voice Hearer

A person that hears voices (sees images, feels sensations) internally in his head (labeled schizophrenia).

First thing to know if you hear voices

First thing to know if you hear voices, see things, or feel sensations:
If you are a person that hears voices when no one is speaking; sees images and other things you know are not there; or feels sensations; then you must know and understand that you are not crazy. Typically, a majority of doctors with western education would likely label you as schizophrenic, and society would likely label you as crazy.
The function of this book is to explain these things to these sufferers, whom from this page onwards we will call "voice hearers." This book is for them and for other people to understand that they are not crazy, and that the doctors are nearly 100% ignorant of these phenomena. In most cases, what you are suffering from, I venture to guess, is brought about by spirits – some evil, some good, and some indifferent and torture individuals. Actual living entities, that I call spirits, which do all these things that you suffer from. This is step number one in understanding your problem.

The second thing to know when you hear voices

The second thing to know when you hear voices are certain undeniable facts that has to do with the physics of the events.
First, there must be a location where the voice is generated from.
Second, there must be something generating the voice or the sound.
Third, there must be a medium for which the sound goes through.
Starting with these facts, we can start investigations to internally or externally locate the point where these voices or sounds are coming from. The process of locating sounds is fairly simple to do using available technology.
These can be the starting steps to finding out where the voices or sounds are coming from, whether it's inside one's head or not, and then investigating who is responsible for the act—perhaps these are small beings or spirits who generate these sounds. With the revelations, a new era can begin. Understanding voice hearers (schizophrenics) will be a revolution in psychiatry and psychology, as well as in religious and social understanding about the spirits, their locations and the gateways to them. The process of controlling these evil spirits and beings can begin. Naturally, we want the good beings and spirits to flourish. In either case, human beings can begin to take control of the invisible world that has controlled or interfered with their life.

So let the process of investigation begin. And here, we can use more engineers than psychiatrists. A new era will begin, one like nothing we know or experienced. The world of the spirits will be revealed. Intelligence, courage, and understanding should push you on this path. The revelations will be plenty, but they must happen. The world of the spirits has and continues to cause human suffering, and I am one of those that suffered and is still suffering. I will not put up with this.

Few know the degree of suffering that these evil spirits can cause a human being especially once his spirit immune system breaks down. It is torture that is unimaginable, that destroys a person's life, and one which continues day and night. And because these people do not know what their condition is, and accept uneducated medical diagnosis that labels them as crazy (schizophrenic), the sufferer becomes more helpless in finding solutions and support, and suffers terribly in silence. To make things worse, the sufferer also has to live with the shame and social stigma that surround this problem. One way to win over this situation is to understand your condition and to explain it to others so that you will not suffer in silence.

Understand your condition and explain it to others, so that you will not suffer in silence

Understand your condition and explain it to others so that you will not suffer in silence. Know that these evil spirits prey on your shame and fear of being ostracized by society. It is like a child that is being raped all the time but does not tell anyone because of shame of being ostracized. Or someone with a terrible disease that he or she wants to hide. The attackers, the evil spirits, know this. They capitalize on it. But like many things, when the light is shone upon the person, evil doers hide or run away. But with silence and darkness, they grow stronger and torture you and me all the more.

These evil spirits harass me and try to rape me while I walk on the streets, sit in both public and private places, while I try to sleep, when I try to have sex with a woman, while I use the toilet, when I'm about to laugh, when I'm happy - almost at every moment of my life. Can you understand this? Can you imagine the effect and the possible results that this can have on the mind, the whole nervous system, the psyche, and the physical body?

These spirits have imprisoned me, beaten me up in my captivity, and continuously tried to rape me at the same time. Can you even begin to comprehend such evilness, my horror and suffering? I can write an entire book if I wanted to say more about this. Such unimaginable suffering!

I met few people who experienced the same torture. One man I met in Hong Kong shared with me his experiences that are similar with mine. I also met people in Thailand and the Philippines who told me about their terrible experience—one that they rather keep a secret. Few speak about this in public, but one person who may have experienced somewhat similar things is a famous singer from the town of Akron, Ohio. Once she dared to tell a radio station about "sleeping with ghosts." I assume she meant it being non-consensual. I met her once at her restaurant but I did not have the presence of mind to ask her about her experience. Still, I encourage others to speak publicly about their experiences so that, hopefully, we can gain desirable results from the new understanding I am providing.

Understand your problem:
The body has an immune system that modern medicine is aware of. White blood cells attack foreign matters such as harmful bacteria, viruses, or fungi. Normally, the body has a huge number of these beings on and in it. The numbers and variety is hard to imagine. Millions and millions of bacteria and other things live on our skin, inside our stomachs and digestive system, inside our mouth, and so on. A healthy person can host these entities without problem. They can also do useful functions sometimes. A normal person does not usually know of the presence of these organisms, or feel anything from them. But when these beings get out of control, or when the body's immune system suffers damage, then these beings can cause sickness to the body.
Similarly, the body has a spirit immune system whose function is to deal with and control spirits that are already inside the body, or those coming from outside. And when this system breaks down, these spirits begin to torture or do other things to humans. Psychiatrists, in ignorance, call schizophrenia. This is the problem. You are not delusional if you hear voices, see images, or feel weird body sensations. Most likely, spirits are doing this to you.
So now, the new science should be locating these small beings, controlling or destroying them!

Of course I have knowledge that you do not have. I am connected to the spirit world, though not by choice. But that is how it is, and you can learn from my suffering. Lotus Sutra explains that Buddha was guided by spirits and he interacted with them. But his particular attention to voice hearers seemed to have gone out of notice and may have been looked upon as a gateway into the spirit world, instead of being an act of love for those suffering. At least for me, I will concede that one publication of an organization that cares about this subject did guess that a long time ago, it was a normal event for people to hear voices, and that this phenomenon seemed to have disappeared with time (from the Australian organization of Hearing Voices investigating this phenomenon). Humans have many hidden capabilities that, intentionally or not, have atrophied with time. When 1200 monks assembled for the Buddha's birthday without being told to do so, it was more than a special day for him. It was a telling story for the whole world, and a revelation to all humans, about mankind's hidden capabilities.

Voice hearers suffer constant voice commentary

Many voice hearers suffer constant voice commentary. They may or may not recognize the voice. Some voices insult them constantly while others may try to help and guide them. Other voices talk to them in a grandiose way about the hearer being a very important figure and that it is time they play their historic role.

Day and night they can be tortured with constant commentary, insults, or meaningless talk, sometimes with images or sensations that make the person's life unbearable to the point of some becoming completely dysfunctional, even leading some to want to commit suicide. Stigma and the lack of understanding from anyone, from family, friends, strangers, or doctors, make their life even more miserable.

Voice hearers need engineers not psychiatrists

Voice hearers need engineers not psychiatrists. Engineers ask the question, "What is going on here?" There are voices that these people hear, there are sounds. Who or what is generating these sounds? What is the source? What is the transmission method used? How frequent is it? What type of frequency? What type of waves? Those suffering do not need psychiatrists giving them drugs that turn them into zombies. Drugs that are based in statistics, not facts. Put 1000 different chemical solutions, give it to mice, and see which one may help. Without any understanding of the underlying mechanisms of the medicine or the damaging side effects, voice hearers continue to suffer. Engineers, please help us! Look into these issues.

Maybe the general knowledge about bacteria used to be unknown. Then more recently, they discovered antibiotics to kill the bad bacteria. Few years later, they discovered something even smaller, the viruses, and then they could see them. That is amazing. Now, time to look for possibly even smaller things, the spirits, and then find a cure for the bad ones. We should get over the wow factor and just focus on finding those beings.

We need engineers to analyze this problem, not voodoo doctors and scientists. Help those people whose suffering is great! Help!

The Third Eye, a place that houses some types of spirits

The third eye seems to be a place that houses good spirits that are related to our most precious connections to the spirit world.

Humans undergo rituals whose origin or meaning they may have already forgotten. Hindus put a red dot in the middle of their forehead, while some Jews put a cube in the same place. Some Christians may mark the same spot in church sometimes. The Buddha is almost always portrayed with a dot in the middle of his forehead eyebrows, the same spot as what the Buddhist Diamond Sutra speaks of as the third eye. I think these are all pointers or reminders of things that have to do with the third eye.

The third eye, which is connected to the spirit world, houses spirits and is linked to parts of the brain that sees inner spirits. This is part of our natural ability, an aspect of what we are capable of. The ancient Egyptians seem to have known this extremely well with their description and depiction of the Eye of Horus, representing and pointing to the exact internal location of the Third Eye inside the brain—somewhere near the thalamus and other nearby structures, such as the pineal gland. Thus, this eye extends from the middle of the forehead to the Thalamus area. Though there may be a strong relationship, I do not know the relation between hearing voices and seeing things, and the Third Eye malfunctioning or being violated and misused by evil spirits. When you look in these areas, it is important to understand that the spirits can be still inside the body, or move, and they can see you first when you are trying to look at them, also, that a whole universe of them can be extremely small! So how can you see one spirit, and you do not even know what its shape is, and as possibly a pure electromagnetic entity. But we must look and find them.

The human body is attuned to many types of fields: electric, magnetic, and gravitational

It is very interesting that a woman's menstrual cycle coincides with the lunar cycle. For the planet to have such a dramatic effect on a human being and in one of their most important body systems, the reproductive system, signifies a significant connection between human beings and the planets. It also has other implications such as the body seemingly attuned to electric, magnetic, and gravitational fields with specific body parts, just like antennas (at macro- and sub-cell level). Incidentally, many religions now follows the lunar cycle, or have started to do so, such as modern Buddhism, Islam, and other old religions.

More knowledge about spirits

You see the world with your eyes, but spirits can see differently. For example, when you enter a building, you may see a person in your direct line of sight. Other spirits in you can see through your peripheral vision or see all around you. Others can see anyone in the entire building. It is not good for humans not to know this. The spirit system is designed to benefit you without your knowledge. However, awareness of this is very important. Now, with the construction of modern tools, remote communication and remote vision between people is common, and is analogous to the biological-spirit system. So when you enter a building with a cellphone at hand, you have the capability to know the presence and proximity of all the people there (if permission is granted). This is like seeing on the phone the presence of your friends nearby, or anywhere! Some spirits may see all the beings in the entire building, while others, in an entire city, etc. In religion (specifically stated in the sutras), the Buddha, after obtaining enlightenment and his special eye, "scanned" to see where some people were, whether in Deer Park or not, etc. In Jain religion, you can obtain such vision when you become a Tirthankara (highest monk).

What this merely means is that a special spirit can come to provide the vision to you or the spirit that is already inside you can awaken and begin to provide this function. This experience is similar to someone handing you a camera with night vision, or infrared vision. The camera shows a part of vision (frequency range) that normally you cannot see.

Extremely important task that all voice hearers should consider

I put this note on my to-do agenda:
Go to the University engineering departments and ask engineers to monitor (using maybe ultrasound, etc.) my head (ear canal, my body, etc.), my surroundings, and walk with me to observe these talking spirits (and later monitor their normal communications when these spirits talk to each other in the same person or between people, and for me, to even walk with me to see what I see when flying spirits bother me in public). Very quickly, one smart engineer is going to realize something and say, "Hey! There may be something to this. I have nothing to lose, and there is earth shaking news to make of this if this is true." But more importantly, you will be helping an untold number of suffering humans. Get the courage. Break the stigma related to this problem, and inform others about and ask for solutions.

My own trial and error in desperation and ignorance

I noticed that when I used a magnet these spirits seem to have been affected. This may be a clue. Try using a magnet to look at the magnetic field before and after a magnet is introduced in order to see the difference. Using many magnets at the same time in the physical areas inhabited by spirits seem to dramatically help in relieving suffering caused by these spirits. Some of these spirits seem to be able to affect the skin directly by creating specific electric or magnetic fields that induce specific sensations, etc. Thus, putting magnets on my shoulders or massaging the area with them, or placing them near my testicles or crotch areas during sleep provided great comfort many times. Also using a simple tone frequency generator software program on my cell phone and sweeping frequencies between 1 to 22,000 HZ (only available range, even though I wanted subsonic frequency ranges and others) for 30 seconds, for example, seemed to have dramatic effects sometimes. Experimenting with sine wave, or square wave, saw tooth wave, etc., made a very noticeable difference. Then later, I used two phones at the same time, running the same software program with frequencies sweeping in phase with the other phone, and this produced more dramatic effects. But I did not know which particular frequency or which scanning produced the results. I am one person with very limited resources and abilities, and was trying things in desperation. Sound frequencies can greatly affect mosquitos, mice, flies, rats, and even break crystal glass. This can also dramatically annoy or injure human ears or serve as a hypnotizer. So maybe some of the frequencies can do the same to some types of spirits. Also, I noticed that using the solfeggio frequencies can have an effect that may not be direct so I could not quantify or qualify. I merely mention this to give you motivation to get started with your search. Sugar was extremely effective in blocking the path of spirits, where they seem to disappear if a sugar bag was in their path. I puzzled and still do over this and do not know the reason if related to the molecular weight, frequency and characteristics of the sugar molecule, and the resulting effects. These should possibly be investigated. Ice was extremely effective when I saw spirits come out of my nose draining from the third eye, I thought, to be attracted to ice and freeze. It was dramatic. I do not have explanations for this.

must add: Magnets seem very effective in repelling or attracting spirits. But adding vibration to the magnets amplified the effectiveness dramatically (by adding a small handheld massage vibrator). It seems that a vibrating electromagnetic field can expose and effect electromagnetic objects much more. If in electrical engineering, an "impulse" can be used to reveal the hidden nature and composition of an electric circuit, a vibrating complex shaped, or magnets (such as two magnets vibrating and moving around each other randomly to change their combined shape, and thus their combined electromagnetic field) can reveal the presence of these spirits or effect them, even if they are hidden or cannot be seen because of their complex nature. Also, other good spirits may have a chance to see them. It is like spraying anti insect chemical spray, where you may not know where they are, but if in the room, they will likely be effected or dye. The EM field will penetrate or disturb the surface or structure outside or inside.

Shapes and forms in the spirit world

In the spirit world, life shapes and forms seem to be continuous in range. That is, just like on a computer where you can design any shape and feature instantly, draw it and have it morph, it is the same in the spirit world where spirits that are in pure electromagnetic non-solid state can be designed and brought to life easily. So if they needed a spirit with 100 legs, they can easily to do it. Other features are meant for traveling in space, or morphing like a cloud, or a flock of birds or school of fish. Some can become a familiar form, like a particular animal, while others can take a completely novel shape.

Locations of these spirits / beings torturing you

I said previously that "voice hearers (schizophrenia) need engineers not psychiatrists". Engineers analyze problems analytically. If there is a sound, there must be: (1) a source to the sound, (2) something the sound is composed of (words and conversations from pressure sound waves or in electromagnetic waves, etc.) and, (3) a medium for the sound to travel through. So starting with the first question, the source can be in the ear, internal or external, or along ear pathway systems (not just nerve pathways, but other body systems also), from the gland at the base of the brain, or from the spine, or all the way from the lower spine, all the way to the pathways leading to the tip of the sexual organs. All along this long pathway, especially the spinal fluid area and areas between the legs, can be an area where these beings live. And when you find these spirits, you can ask them questions about their world and yours (how they see it). But the engineers have to find them, and not the other way around. When this happens, the relationship between humans and spirits is on equal terms, and we can communicate directly and clearly as humans communicate with each other, not using voodoo methods. This will then open the door to the spirit world. Otherwise, until engineers develop the needed tools, this door should remain closed and not be opened. Technology as far as I know is our one and only salvation to overcome this situation.

We need to see the evil spirits under the microscope, and control them directly or at least not allow them to control us, and not have to deal with voodoo religions, cultures, and beliefs. We need to be in charge of our own destiny and not be at their mercy.

Here is a dilemma. You are looking for something that does not want to be found. They are extremely smart, aware of you, your thoughts and actions! And some are part of your creation. As you look for them, they already know what you think, where you will look, and worse, they will be the ones leading you to false alleys and to change direction or to stop this search, with their function as part of your thought process. So it is a very difficult task. But every now and then things change, and opportunities open, because other spirits have different views and want people to know of this world, and that the two worlds are connected intimately and work together, and it is improper to use the size advantage to treat human as children when they are an integral part of a common life, with spirits living in people, and many of are from relatives, and care greatly about the person, such as the spirit of a dead mom or father or grandma, or the holy spirit which has a special protector role similar in some ways to the role white blood cells play in protecting you from bacteria or viruses etc.

Example 1: Sound Waves

Firecracker is burned somewhere unknown.

Sound waves are generated

→

Technical Equipment 1 kilometer away Hears the sound, and determines exact location of the sound.

Firecrackers are located. People lighting the firecrackers are located, and catched.

Example 2: Electromagnetic Waves

Cell phone is stolen and used somewhere unknown.

Electromagnetic waves are generated

→

Technical Equipment hundreds of kilometers away Detect the waves, and determines exact location of the wave source.

Phone is located. People using the phone are located, and catched.

Helping Patients   ....   Transforming Psychiatry Into a Science

Example 3:

Sound is heard inside a patient's mind

Internal firecracker sound is heard inside patient's head.

Sound waves
or
electromagnetics waves
or
chemical messenger molecules are generated to carry the wave from unknown source to unknown destination (internal ear of patient) Using an unknown medium or pathway for the transmission

→

Technical Equipment to detect sound location cannot be placed inside the patient's internal ear to hear the sound.

And we do not know the exact spot for the internal ear if we could insert the equipment or an electric probe, or non-invasive probe

Therefore, the sound source cannot be located.

How do we solve this problem?

What are available options?

Do we take a completely different approach than this traditional method of sound location?

↓

If we can solve this problem, we would have solved the first and big part of the puzzle. The second part then becomes catching the source generating the sound from this spot. These creatures are extremely tiny. But the task should be achievable.
Our problem is solved. The patient can be helped by destroying the source, convincing it not to harrass the patient, other options available.

We are two legged from birth

We are two legged from birth, and our body is straight from birth. However, since the legs are not strong enough at birth to hold the body up, and the baby is difficult to hold in the womb for more than 9 months to develop such strength, the baby comes out and must walk on feet and hands for a short while. When the baby does this, bad things seem to happen to it. These bad things happen because of how the spirit world functions in relations to humans. In general, when you perform an activity, a spirit master (lord, group leader, or whatever it may be called) issues you a spirit associated with this skill that becomes part of you. This spirit takes over or assists in the skill you are learning or have learned. So when a baby walks on feet and hands, he receives an animal spirit for walking in a manner similar to animals, and with this unwanted gift, which must be accepted, humans fall under the power of this spirit which becomes dominant in human life because it is one of the earliest spirits received and becomes a leading and primary spirit in all of a human being's life. This spirit should be removed from the body. Alternatively, although not a good option because it is limiting, the child may not be allowed to walk on hands and feet. The child would first walk upright with help of baby carriage. I do not know if the spirit received in this case is from the animal world, or from the human world for simply walking on hands and feet without the need of association with animal behaviors and instincts. An aside: this spirit world functions in parallel with our physical being world, and these spirits live in that world, and, eventually, as we get older, become more and more dominant in taking on normal functions control. Finding these spirit centers in the body is important for better control of our destiny. These spirits force codependency on them. They are an interjection from the spirit world to become in control. I think they are not needed and their intervention and assistance is better not wanted. The body has many control centers or pathways to a center that controls a function or all functions. Some of these centers are called Chakra centers in some religions or cultures.

Explaining a voice hearer (schizophrenia) problem to others is like talking to a wall

To begin with, it is so difficult and frustrating for a voice hearer to talk about their problem. First there is tremendous social stigma. So typically, they will not tell anyone about their problem, and therefore their problem will be compounded by lack of help from others.

But worse even, is that when they muster the courage to talk about their problem, they find out that explaining their problem to others can be like talking to a wall. Normal people have no such experience in the voice hearing realm, and therefore, it is extremely difficult for them to understand this strange world of the voice hearer and their suffering. It is better for voice hearers to tell others about their problem, and find smart ways to explain their suffering and experience so that others can understand and help.
Shine the light on these evil spirits that win because of darkness. This darkness is the evil doers' weapon. Shine the light so we can win.

How to help those who suffer hearing voices, seeing things, feeling things, schizophrenia

How to help those who suffer hearing voices, seeing strange things, feeling strange things? Many things are needed, and they all may not be enough, but some help is better than no help sometimes. And even if the problem does not go away, it is important to help lower the level of suffering. This can make a big difference in the quality of life for these people.
First, listen to them in order to understand their problem.
Do not be judgmental. Their problem is real and they cannot control it.
Ask them questions and show real understanding and care.
Give love and support, by looking for things that make them happy, and give these things to them. Things such as music (listening to it or attending a concert), tasty drink or cup of tea, a tasty meal, a subject they like to talk about to engage them with, a walk to physically get them moving. You can also help take them to gym to exercise. Touching and caressing and lots of massages are so important. Take them to social events to keep them interacting with others. The real fight starts when their spirit immune system (a system similar to a white blood cell immune system) gets strong from good smells and tastes, nice imagery, active physical activity, and relaxing and enjoyable time. Or when they are surrounded by good and caring people. That is how you can help treat this sometimes unbelievably severe problem while we try to find a real cure to these evil or malfunctioning spirits torturing them. Every time a suffering person feels good even for one moment, their well-being and internal fighting system gets stronger, and the evil spirits loose. But the bottom line is that you are helping a suffering person feel better, even if it is just for one moment.

Group help

Meditation, in addition to normal use of better self-control, can be used to remove or control bad spirits, probably best with group meditation, praying and chanting and asking good spirits for this to happen. Meditation with eyes ¾ closed looking down, as you see the Buddha statue in meditation, may be a good position and door to enter the world between wake and sleep, for meditation. Just as laying of hands, which I am fairly certain is helpful and can be effective, so is surrounding a suffering person, with loving and caring people to lay hands, and touch, and surround in a powerful posture as if the person is being physically protected from a present evil force. Group power, when focused on an individual, and in a prolonged and repeated way, may be extremely effective way to help those suffering hearing voices, and what today is called schizophrenia. Three, five, 10, 20 or 30 or more people who have clean spirits, and are caring, when circling a suffering person, touching the person in a loving and supportive way, for a long period, and praying for him or doing acts or words of support are important.

Engineers, just take a look

I said that voice hearers (schizophrenia) need engineers not psychiatrists. In order to help locate the source of the voice, (later the images or sensations) and who or what is generating these conversations or statements that those who are suffering hear.
Let me help a little in the search effort. These are things I already know with certainty (based on my experience), while other things I know with fair degree of certainty, and other things as speculation. But first I have to tell engineers these technically inclined facts as preparation.
1. As computers got smaller over the years, they got faster, more efficient, packed more memory. And this trend continues for silicon chips based computers. So the smaller the chip (and its transistors), the better it can be. In the future we will build very tiny computers, and because of this, they can be better. So to say that spirits are very small beings, should not sound strange. The smaller, can mean the faster and better, and possibly more intelligent.

2. When you listen to traditional over-the-air radio, for example, you can be hundreds or thousands of kilometers away from the radio station and its broadcast tower, yet, you and millions of people can listen to this radio (electromagnetic signal) at the same time, even if the people are very widely spread apart. What is important to note from this is that the electromagnetic signal can touch all these people and fill all this space without any problem and do it instantly. Now, I can suggest you look also for electromagnetic signal as not only a transmission method for these spirits, but also as the construction structure of these spirits. That is, some if these beings are made from electromagnetic structure. Transistors can be made from silicon, some of these beings are made from electromagnetic fields/components. Imagine how fast, and intelligent, and how their body can touch a wide area or many things at the same time and widely spread apart. This understanding can have further ramifications, and benefits in learning about many useful things, but I merely focus on these evil spirits. Not commercial or scientific benefits which can be enormous. Warning, and a big warning: some spirits have additional properties and are living beings, just like humans, some good, or many are good, some evil, and some indifferent. The range of spirits can be unimaginable for us as I am opening an area that I am not aware there is any knowledge about. Some of these spirits are very connected to

us, came from our families, are with us since birth, others related to the hidden world that religion talks about, and others are about animal spirits, or robotic ones . So how do you know the good spirits from the evil ones in this search for their locations, where some spirits are very dear to us, or consider holy (because they are related to creation, or our protection, or the system at large), etc.? This question must be contemplated, as our world will not be the same from such encounters. But the spirits torturing human beings, should be easy to identify, from the communication and act. I believe good spirits will guide and help guide because they want to, or because of necessity to avoid being hurt themselves in this process (just like targeting cancer cells area with radiation can destroy nearby good cells in the process). Maybe all this was meant to be secret, and for the better, and maybe it is better if there is transparency and these two worlds connect. I don't know the consequences. But here it is I am telling it to you. Have reverence and care for a world unknown to you, but known to me, and I hope future lives will be better. Volumes can be written in science and religion about what will open up, so again, reverence because they are part of you and life. True or not, it said in the Bible "man was created in god/gods image" and _all_ is yours except one tree, to stay away from, else you become like gods. That was a warning, from loving creators, I think, not from jealousy. I do not know the consequences well, but this is not a commercial venture, but simply trying to solve one problem that may solve many other problems also, in the human realm and the spirit realm. Things I cannot explain now.

An aside: Some of these spirits I encountered can naturally communicate by light projection. Projection of images and video. Just like a human typically uses a pen to write words or speak them, these spirits can write images and videos spontaneously as means of communication. Their ability seems extremely high and I am not able to quantify it or qualify it.

What kind of suffering these people have
They have voices talking to them. Commanding them sometimes. Telling them a wide range of evil things nonstop, such as "kill yourself", or "your sister is being raped now", etc. they often talk nonstop, preventing the person from being able to concentrate on any task. Therefore, it effects their entire life dramatically, family, work, study, relations, social life, health, etc.
Some are bothered as they try to sleep with voices or images that are scary or annoying so as to prevent them from falling asleep. Some experience horrible nightmares, sleep paralysis and being raped in their dreams or while in different stages of sleep cycle. The spirits torture and try to take control. If a person does not sleep, their next day is affected. They will be tired, and less focused and less energetic. Day after day, the results

accumulate, and again, it becomes any additional method for these spirits to weaken, control or destroy this person. Lack of sleep eats away at your body and mind.

Some sufferers smell odors, when there are none. They smell an apple or bad odors, such as bad toilet odors, etc.

Some see images, still or animated, when eyes are open or closed.

Some experience strange or unwanted physical feelings, such as being touched on different parts of your body, and sometimes sexual areas. Some can be raped while awake, with or without body paralysis. Some may feel animals crawling on them etc. Incidentally, that is why these sufferers often do not tell anyone about their problem because they are embarrassed and because of social stigma and because of lack of understanding by others when they are told. They tend to think it is all imaginary in the mind of the sufferer. They do not understand these are real phenomena. Even the sufferers themselves do not understand what is causing these phenomenon. They do not know it is actual beings, spirits, which are torturing them. And it also **involves spirit sexual and rape rituals.** Like a bad bacteria or virus or fungus in your system: it needs to be controlled or destroyed to stop their acts. Intentional, conscious acts!!!! The suffering is so severe that many consider or try suicide.

Is severe depression or anxiety related to spirits also?

I would like to stay much focused in on voice hearers (labeled by today's western medicine as schizophrenia). But to help also these sufferers of severe depression and severe anxiety, the answer can be yes: spirits are involved in this sometimes. But these can be not evil spirits torturing you as in schizophrenia, but rather good spirits that normally help you, and are being tortured themselves, or they are worried about you or your future. These spirits are strongly connected to you and care about you, and when you are in severe crisis, or they anticipate problems coming your way in the future, they can be stressed, and this will weaken your support system, your spirits support system, and rational worries about life encountered problems of love, or money, or health, turn into severe depression or severe anxiety, which can be debilitating and life destroying problem, leading many to even think or attempt suicide. Severe depression and severe anxiety are the flip side of schizophrenia, good spirits being concerned, but in some cases, the same side of schizophrenia, evil spirits involved.

In problems such as so-called Bipolar, it can be a combination of spirits sinking you into depression while others after lifting you out quickly. **Some spirits may have direct access to physical centers in the brain concerned with these areas, while others may have access to the pathways,** still others can reach or effect these areas very indirectly such as X-Rays, MRIs, and ultrasound can reach certain spots in the body without being intrusive.

You can touch an area in the brain directly by an electric probe, or indirectly by waves, ultrasound, electromagnetic, magnetic, etc. That same area can also be touched or controlled along the systems that connect to it such as the nerve system. These nerves are leading to it in the brain, and some, continue to outside the brain such as the spine and rest of the body. So from the spine areas, or skin areas, you can touch or effect these brain centers or parts. With this said, we should dispose of modern psychiatry and quack spirit traditional medicine (even though some traditional medicine people or normal people are connected to the spirit world and can be great help), for engineering based psychiatry. We scan for alien life using equipment that looks at millions of frequencies at the same time into outer space to detect signs of intelligence. Now, simply look no further than centimeters away from you or in you to find them. It will still be a difficult task, because you are dealing with extremely intelligent life forms, and some are watching you in the lab while doing this!, but understand that this is life in a good way, and if some of it was meant to be a secret, it is with **the best of intentions, right or wrong. Worth noting that if you are intelligent, the tiny single cell that created you, and its much tinier genetic code may have more intelligence and is the one that gave you your intelligence. So spirits may be in them, or on them, or trying to control them remotely.**

Rape in dreams

Few days ago, I met a lady that often has dreams, unwanted dreams, of having sex with her father. She feels dirty, troubled mentally, because she has no control over dreams. She feels ashamed and does not tell her father or mother about her dreams. She is an adult, and her father apparently is a good father and does no such acts to her in real life. I have had sexual nightmares myself also, of different types. Also, almost every night, I go to sleep, with fears of such nightmares and other types, and I experience visual harassment that try to prevent me from sleeping. I have met others with similar problems. Some have sleep paralysis with spirits and beings on them or around them. Others wake up trying to fight rape attempts.

These spirits that cause these dreams, do this, because they are evil. They want us to suffer. And to not sleep and be tired and dysfunctional from lack of sleep and fatigue. And to put us in a downward negative cycle, of fatigue, of lack of ability to concentrate, and of weakness of body and mind. All these can make us more and more vulnerable to these spirits and their control.

I do not know the immediate answers or solution to this. I can only think of finding these spirits to kill or control them. However, this is not within our technological medical grasp yet so we need to ensure that we do not take drugs or alcohol as this may weaken the physical and spiritual immune system, and make the problem worse. We need to prevent unhealthy things from going into our body and mind. Unhealthy things such as unhealthy foods, unhealthy images and videos and films, unhealthy smells, unhealthy music, and unhealthy touch, etc. We need to try to watch beautiful nourishing videos and movies and images that makes us happy, and laugh. These are the things that we need to do instead of watching sad movies, or movies and images of violence, or other unwholesome activities. We need to eat delicious food that nourish the body and senses. Listen to uplifting music that gives us energy and happiness, instead of things that depress us. We need to have an environment that smells good. Be around good friends and good environment (parks, museums, etc.) and social events that pull us to do wholesome activities, instead of pulling us into bad activities such as drugs, drinking, violence, unwholesome sex, unhealthy movies, etc.). It is good to exercise to stay healthy and in good shape. Dance, take walks, have sex if you are of proper age. Sex is a great release for the body and mind, feels great, and is another very strong activity when done in wholesome ways to help distract from the pain and inability to focus (which voice hearers suffer from). Get massages to relax the body, and relieve stress. The sense of touch is so important to be nourished. Meditate to relax, empty, and control your mind. In essence, any activity that feels good, distract the mind from the evil spirits' chatter or images or sensations, so that the person can gain momentary focus, should be attempted if possible, and these activities help create moments of nourishment and rest for the mind and its good spirits, to collect themselves, to feel good, restore their energy, so that the person can fight back this severe problem, and meantime, also have moments of joy in his/her life, so that no matter the outcome, the person is being helped to optimize his life despite a very difficult and, possibly, a prolonged situation.

We need to speak out about our problems and not hide them. By speaking to caring people to let others know our situation, even though this can be very difficult in some societies, or in some families. When a person has these kinds of very difficult mental sufferings (labeled by some doctors as schizophrenia), those people suffering and their human support system need to do all these steps to help their body and mind fight these evil spirits that are causing the suffering. This may not be a complete solution, but it may lessen the problem, and help eventually lead to recovery. When a person is suffering, every little step to make the problem less, may be a very good thing to do. Don't feel guilty about your situation, because it is not of your own making, or under your control. When evil spirits torture you and try to destroy your life, the answer can be to try to do the opposite, to try to enjoy life as much as you can in a healthy way. This can be the best medicine to enhance your physical and mental immunity, so that you can have the will and energy to fight back and live, and hopefully, have happiness in your difficult life.

How do you explain to your psychiatrist and normal people what is going on?

If you hear voices that are bothering you, inside your head, effecting and interfering in your life, or see images awake or while eyes closed, or have bodily sensations, how do you explain it to your psychiatrist, let alone a normal human being who has no experience or understanding in these areas?

First of all, the number one issue I know from meeting people suffering from these problems is that they themselves do not have an explanation for what is happening to them, and why, and what to do about it. They hear voices, and the public usually may label them as "crazy" or "going crazy", so that is the limit of their understanding in western cultures and many cultures. There are exceptions (such as true Hindu or true Buddhist cultures). And when they go to a psychologist or psychiatrist, they are almost certainly diagnosed and labeled as schizophrenic, which means little more that the person hears internal voices, etc. There is no understanding of the problem—the underlying problem and the cause. The person is "suffering from evil spirits that have access to these bodily facilities of hearing, or vision system, or sensation system, etc. So the person suffering does not know, and neither does the doctor. I am shedding a new light on this problem, telling the real causes, and this will meet with fantastic disbelief, and cynicism, but the task is to educate sufferers, doctors, and the public about this. Similar to the time when people and some of supposed all-knowing churches in ancient history taught and believed that the earth was flat, and imprisoned scientists for saying otherwise, later found out the earth is round. I am saying, these people do not have a brain malfunction, that makes the brain produce sounds, images, or sensations, randomly, or otherwise, the problem is that our world is full of spirits, good, indifferent, and the evil ones that are doing these acts. Similar to a virus attack on the body, or bacterial attack or presence with the immune system compromised or malfunctioning, these are conscious acts by spirits in typically against a human being.

The very difficult part is explaining to anyone that there are spirits, that these spirits are unbelievable abundant, and they are all around us, and in us, and normally we are not aware of them, until something severely wrong happens. Most people on earth reportedly believe in a god, and have a religion that they accept. What is remarkable in my experience is that few of these people tend to ask themselves the important questions, such as "if there is a god, if there are angels, if people when they die they go to a different world, then are these beings not spirits, that is, non-biological beings?" Then, if there are such beings, and I will call them generally spirits, then those religious people have to accept the existence of spirits. Jesus in the Bible is said to have cast out evil spirits from people. The Buddha almost always interacted with the spirits in the sutras. Hindu Vedas talk about humans being spirits inhabiting body. And it goes on for other religions. So why does a Christian psychiatrist not believe the bible and that there are evil spirits in the body, and that Christ cast them out. Or that a Buddhist psychiatrist not believe spirits are the cause when the Buddhist sutras are full of the Buddha interacting with spirits, good and bad. Similarly, why does a Hindu not believe the Vedas? Aside from all this, and more importantly, you do not know me, and I do not care, what is important is what is being said, and if possibly logical or at all possible, and what I care to tell you is that I know these are spirits, I see them with my eyes, I can hear them and interact with them, etc. It is not delusional, or a brain malfunction, etc. The Hindu Vedas, speak of such interaction. The Buddha sutras are absolutely full of such interaction. Jesus cast the evil ones out, and at the well, told the lady about herself, without her telling him personal information. He knew about her personal life. So the earth is not flat, it is round according to these religious teachings. And, schizophrenia is not a brain malfunction, even though in **some few cases physical injury or defects may be a cause**, the problem baring physical defect is evil spirits attacking the brain functions.

In psychology, there is the term "psychological dissonance". It is when a human being holds two conflicting ideas at the same time. For example in this case, some people believe in a particular religion where the religion speaks of the presence of spirits, but these same individuals, if you speak to them outside the field of religion, they will likely say they do not believe spirits exist, or to such an extent, or that they can interfere in human function. These are two opposing ideas, held by the same person. It means something is wrong with your thinking. You either accept the reality of spirits, or you reject your religion. You cannot have both believes at the same time. Same for a Christian, Buddhist or Hindu psychiatrist. If you do not accept these facts, then you suffer psychological dissonance, and as such, you need to resolve this problem in your mind, before you try to help the minds of other people!!!!!! If you care about your own profession, and your patients, you owe it to yourself to open your eyes very wide for new possibilities. Schizophrenia is not a typical brain malfunction, needing medicine, it is evil spirits attacking or manipulating brain centers and functions directly or from the nerves system or other body systems know or unknown (such as endocrine system or unknown itch system etc.), or even attacking the body at the cell level, anywhere in the body, or even possibly at the DNA messenger or DNA itself. Some of these spirits in my own personal experience demonstrated extreme knowledge of the human body functions at all levels! Many possess great knowledge of all life forms and the life system itself and its connectedness. If life is a conscious creation as I have seen it, or has evolved to this level, this should not be surprising. Let us start the engineering work, to understand the methods of attacks of these spirits, and their forms after, so we can block their attacks first, and locate them next. It is a challenging task, with many dimensions, medical, human, spiritual and religious. But the task has to be done. Humans should not be at the mercy of such evil spirits.

Research efforts are just beginning

Here is one study to identify the problem. But typically, they have no idea what the problem is:

Tuning in to the Voices: A Multisite fMRI (Functional MRI) Study of Auditory Hallucinations

http://www.ncbi.nlm.nih.gov/pmc/articles/PMC2643968/

On the secrets of life, secrets you may never ever come across

I think one of the most important things if not the most important a human being should do is to destroy his karma, from birth, before the spirits start to come into his body at the karma center and nest. I think these spirits come at first breath, and help and control much in your life. It sounds good, but may be very bad. It is like being on strings all your life, and as you grow in age, these spirits grower stronger, doing more of the work, while your own natural thinking faculties atrophy from such invisible dependency. It is like a puppet on a string, controlled in action and direction. Like a robot. It is better you do the thinking etc. A human will grow his own natural visible faculties and hopefully will by this act, not allow spirits to have visible or invisible control of his actions and life. Another benefit is that a human being will not have strong connections to things controlling his life, but he does not understand, and are not under his control. A poor analogy, and I cannot think of a good one now, but somewhat useful analogy, is that before a human is born, he is a literally a physical part a woman's body, and she is in control of the baby's destiny. But upon birth, she forces the baby out and cuts the umbilical cord, and by doing these acts, the baby is now a separate independent body, that can grow on its own, to later become strong and can function on its own. Similarly, severing your karma hosting area in your body, severs your connection to the spirit world, and prevents all kinds of good or parasitic spirits from coming and nesting in your body. This allows a human to become much stronger later, but most importantly, it destroys the control center that spirits come to nest in and control the human being, almost always, completely invisibly and unknowingly to a human. Until we develop the x-ray similar systems to find out and see these locations in the human body, (and animals similarly have them), and be able to control these centers, they should be destroyed. We can have controlled communications later when we develop the technology to connect to the spirit world, in a respectful and intelligent manner, just as two human adults communicate directly with each other and directly seeing each other, even if under an x-ray microscope, not as an unknown being communicating and controlling your life in unknown and unseen manner. There is much more to explain, especially for people who do not know what a karma is, or if it actually exists, and if there are spirits, and if they actually live in or on your body, etc... I have to explain this later here or on my other blogs. Every now and then a comet can come to earth with new material, or a more powerful telescope gives greater view of the universe or a stronger microscope gives deeper view into inner space to atoms and beyond for new discoveries. If what I say makes sense then please spread the word. I am asking for your help, not to believe, but to think and to let others think, and hopefully know.

Hearing Voices Organization

I do not remember the exact date, but roughly around 15 years ago, about 4 years after my experience with the spirit world began, important information about the world I was experiencing and explanations for it did not exist as per my extensive research. I needed help and explanation. The few that existed were practically useless in understanding, depth, or practicality. And to think that this happened while I was living in the USA and in the age of internet. No books were available. One organization, called Hearing Voices, which is based in Australia, stood out not because of its knowledge base, but because of its effort to help and understand the problem. It is also worth mentioning that they were able to produce the only book on the subject. The book spoke about research efforts (as well as research results) aimed to understand this phenomena. It had no details about the reality of this subject, but it was useful in the sense that it reassured people who have similar experiences with hearing voices. Sometime last year, I decided I needed to go public with my experience and knowledge, and looked up the organization website briefly. Despite this, I failed to see anything publicly listed that was interesting and useful. My search also showed poor results. So I sent a voice recorded email to important research centers in psychiatry around the world to educate them a little and to get the ball rolling so-to-speak. Emails to Harvard, Oxford, Yale, etc. I requested privacy. I did not get any response back, or saw relevant results. I hope my new book will be useful and promoted heavily by thoughtful people to start what is nothing short of a new revolution in understanding our world, and how to solve spirits-related problems, as well as to advance technology. It will be a new chapter in recorded history as I know it.

The veil between heaven and earth

In Buddhism there are stories about the robe that a monk wears. I will make my own version of the robe story. A most or the most important question for some who knows of earth and heaven is if the robe, when worn, should reveal the left or right shoulder. For those not connected to the spirit world, the language can seem strange and incomprehensible, and sometimes intentionally, as the preserve of those who know. But if you think of the left shoulder as the left side of the brain and right shoulder as the right side of the brain, then the symbolism is revealed and a new meaning can be understood. It seems logical that a Buddhist monk robe should hang on the right shoulder or the left, to reveal only one side, otherwise, the robe will fall down, revealing the whole. This is a great symbolism. And maybe most appropriate for its time. The right side of the brain, supposedly according to modern science is the conscious mind, and the left side the unconscious. What modern science does not know is the connection of the left side to the heavens, that is, the spirit world that is not revealed or understood. This is the domain of religion, spirits, and the few monks who are greatly or lightly connected to it. So with this book, I am revealing important parts of the left side, which in time should unravel the rest of this world. It is most appropriate now to reveal the right and left shoulders letting the robe of shame drop. Ashamed of what?

Saying: I think, maybe

I entered the world of the spirits, a strange world unknown to me before, for the first time. For over some twenty years, I saw many things, and I understood many things, and came to know more things I did not see or understand. I was also told by many spirits about many things. Even when I saw and was told, many times I remained skeptical. I have to tell people about this experience. But how do I do this, and be accurate when I do it? I tried to resort to use of the words "I think" and "maybe" in many sentences, which may make it sound like I am speculating or do not know what I am talking about. In the spirit world, where vision was provided, it is like looking through binoculars, where the images beyond can be real or made up. It is like chatting on the internet with strangers, where you do not know if the being you are talking to is a human or machine, and the video you see is real or made up. Even when I was fairly certain, I could not be 100% certain. So would you rather I tell you nothing about this world or share my experience as best as I can? Or it is like landing on a strange planet. Many strange things and events happened, some I understand and some not. I just report what I saw and what I understood, or thought I understood. This is what I have done.

Politics on earth and life in the spirit world

For me, looking at the overall big political conflicts that have dominated between countries over history, there are the conflicts started by self-interest, or as a power grab of the strong taking over a weaker country to take or use its resources, and other non-ideological reasons. Also, there have been the ideological struggles, and this is what I will focus on. Here, a constant struggle has been between those love freedom and so-called democracy, and those who favor dictatorship and militarism.

Athena and Sparta are used as example from history, while a more recent example is the struggle between the West and the Soviet Union.

The implication for an individual person is what system he will eventually live under: a system that gives him/her the right of choice in all matters, to live according to their own likes, or a system that imposes limits on this person without their consent.

It seems like those who love freedom and fight for it win, but at great cost.

Also it seems, after those who fight on the side of freedom win, internal deterioration takes place because people get lacks about vigilance. So corruptions in the system can spread, and fiefdoms can develop, and the main good ruler or president gets weaker at the expense of many individuals who create their own power centers, or departments, etc. and after a long time of this ongoing corruption, each of these individual will get to think of themselves as the ruler, or equivalent, and together, all the corrupt individuals, who in effect become like a shadow government, get to think that they are the government and rulers.

The true and original ruler in effect is pushed aside, and over a long time, may get to even disappear from the scene and get forgotten. So every rat gets to think of himself as a president or a king. And every department head thinks that nothing can happen without their permit, as the final arbiter. So, the original president/ruler/king becomes ineffective. The system is now corrupt, and very difficult to fix. To get anything done, you have to deal with so many self-appointed and self-dignified officials or persons, that the system can be said to be in chaos, and nearly unfixable. The results can be very ineffective government, gangs and outlaws controlling different parts of government or people's lives.

This has happened so many times in history in so many places, and people can understand this phenomenon.

For example, if a person wanted to get something accomplished, he may need to fight, bribe, beg, request, so many officials, where normally, the process would be clear, simple, and quick.

Other times, when those freedom loving win the fight against dictators, they try to unknowingly create a dictatorship in their own country, but a dictatorship of a different kind, a dictatorship created by the citizens, who start to demand and force creation of laws granting right to education, to health care, to social security, etc. these just demand it, as a right, and want the other rich or not rich citizens to pay for it. As if one rich citizen (or not rich) owes another human being an education, or health care etc. these freedom-uneducated citizens demand confiscating other people's money, through tax laws, for their own benefits. These people fail to see how they are taking the freedom of other citizens. But it seems to be the case that many citizens are not educated enough to understand the result of their seemingly well-motivated desire for a good society. And many politicians and interests play on the uneducated desires, to create a self-perpetuating freedom constricting machine that is hard to dismantle because of the many ill-educated or crooked interests.

From what I know about the spirit world, and it is so much more than the average individual, but I still know very little, I am guessing that the big struggles in the heavens are the same. Those who want freedom and peace, and those who want dictatorship and militarism. Two different approaches to life and solving problems.

And when I see the spirit world now, it is a corrupt system taken over by fiefdoms who have assumed they are the rulers. There is the cat fiefdom and its chief, the mosquito's fiefdom, the bird fiefdom, and the untold kinds of spirits. Each in charge of an area ad the absolute and ultimate dictator of it. Many of these spirit fiefdoms are of animal spirits or animal-like spirits. Still, these spirits are extremely endowed with intelligence in the heaven world, but they do not lose certain basic animal characteristics that keeps them different from human spirits. And these animal spirits, so much outnumber human spirits, that by mere numbers and volume, they have dramatically changed the power structured in the heavens. They have become the power centers and holders. Incidentally, some religions may call these spirits demigods or gods.

Just like on earth, a society may start fresh, with freedom in it flourishing for all, to do as they wish, and not impose on others demands, soon, this society starts to change, and each citizen, with his own ideas, desires to impose on others. Some want to impose how you dress, some want to impose mandatory education, others mandatory health care, etc. They all mean well, but they do not understand the consequences of such thinking. That they are taking away other people's choices or money, without consent. But this argument is difficult to make. Much easier is for the ignorant politicians or crooked ones or special interest to tell the public "we will give you many things, just elect us, and put us in power. We will give you, health care, social security, education, and many other laws you may want us to impose on the public. Just elect us!"

And that is the state of most if not all countries on earth. Corrupt, because freedom has been robbed away from people by uneducated well-meaning intentions, and politicians who prey on this for their own self-interest, or because they are equally uneducated about the consequences of their actions and slogans.

And the result is what we see on earth, of wars between countries, or internally between the people, and creation of fiefdoms, and poor spread of freedom, and even in economically well to-do countries, their status is worse than what it can be.

I speculate this is exactly the case in the heavens. The majority of spirits, which have animal-like Law Of The Jungle, a form of dictatorship of the strong, that sees rape as acceptable way to have sex, because the strong has this right over the weaker one, want to impose their system on human spirits. That of power dictatorship, and restrictions, instead of values of freedom and peace (where people have to consent to others on issues affecting their life).

On earth, animals by a huge-huge margin outnumber people. But we do not let their system (way of life) govern us. We cage them and put them in zoos, despite their enormous physical powers compared to humans. But in the heavens, it has become a different story, the animal-like spirits have slowly taken over. And now, they will be so difficult to dislodge, and restore things to be under control.

Why would a human being make a mistake?

Why would a human being consciously make a mistake? Where is the logic in that? Does a human being set out to make a mistake when a mistake happens? Of course not. Humans do not intentionally make a mistake.

Someone else is doing the mistake. Human beings are blameless! Many spirits are usually inside you.

When humans do wrong, it is because they do not know better. So how can they be blamed? If they knew better, they would be doing what is better, unless their physical wiring or processing is defective or the information is incomplete.

The earth - heaven system is broke

What if there were life forms extremely intelligent and we are unaware of. And these beings were unseen by us. What if these being knew the genetic code of humans, or can decode it. What if these beings can decode any code? If a being can decode the genetic code, would we lose our freedom, in that, they will be able to control us?

Just having an electric probe (electrode) touch the brain in some areas, we can control a human being (or touch him along the spine and other nerve pathways, touching by electric probe, or externally by electromagnetic waves). If there are such beings and they already can do this to us, then how do we preserve our freedom from becoming robots, controlled by them? I know there are such beings that are invisible to us, and are extremely intelligent and can or have access to important parts of our mental and bodily functions. If they already know our body-mind system, and our protection system that is now in place no longer can fight them (our spirit defense system, analogous to the physical white blood cells defense system), the answer is probably to let humans have access to the same information (available in the spirit world), instead of just waiting for humans to discover it in the laboratory. Maybe no such thing was allowed before because there is a separation wall between earth and heaven, so that beings in the heavens, do not interfere in human affairs. This was meant in essence to protect the freedom of humans from these unseen beings. But this separation wall system is broken, and these heavenly beings (evil ones) are interfering in human lives in major ways. And these beings, though very advanced, seem to retain animal like instincts. In short, humans need to know what is going on, and the location of these evil beings, and how to fight them. The task may not be very complicated, since these spirits are around us. We just need proper technical tools to locate them, listen and watch them, and destroy or control them.

It is an engineering problem that may require help from heavenly beings. There are victims sometimes in such major undertakings, and this task is not for everyone to take on. I have been a victim of these evil beings among many voice-hearing sufferers. My life practically has been savagely destroyed by them. I just hope there will not be too many more victims like me, and that the task can be done to destroy or control these beings, and control our own destiny. Voice-hearer are not crazy, imagining things. These are real beings talking to them, and doing other things. These are spirits and some of them are good, some indifferent, and some very evil torturing us.

Supposedly, this system is for the benefit of both, man and spirits

Among the many things I was told and learned from spirits is what one important spirit summarized to me that: the system is designed for the benefit of both of them, spirits, and humans. That is to both exist on equal terms and codependent on each other, and not a master - slave type relationship.

Important key to understanding the Buddhist sutras

I think the most important key to understanding the Buddhist sutras is this: when the Buddha was talking, he frequently is talking about his spirit, about himself as a spirit, not as a flesh human body. When a normal human being talks, he is talking about himself as a flesh body, the person that eats, drinks, etc. when the Buddha is talking, it is about the spirit inside his body. When this is understood, then many if not all the strange statements in the sutras become understandable. So for example, bellow, from the Diamond Sutra, when the Buddha says that the rajah cut every piece of his limbs, he is talking about his spirit being cut into its parts, its limbs, etc.

While a human being would likely be dead from being cut to pieces like that, a spirit has a different type of body, and can survive such acts. It is like an electromagnetic field that you can shop, yet it is capable of maintaining its integrity, or greatly so, or at least for its important parts or functions (or neural brain network, or electronic one, that parts can be damaged, but reconstructs and maintains the data. Same for a functional device that can maintain function even with some damage. This can be an extremely advanced construction method of a tool, and a future consideration in the construction of electromagnetic robots.)

It almost cannot be understood what the Buddha was saying in the many sutras unless you keep in mind that it is a spirit talking about itself, aware that it is a spirit, and talking from this perspective.

From the Diamond Sutra:

Subhuti, the Tathagata teaches likewise that the Perfection of Patience is not the Perfection of Patience: such is merely a name. Why so? It is shown thus, Subhuti: When the Rajah of Kalinga mutilated my body, I was at that time free from the idea of an ego-entity, a personality, a being, and a separated individuality. Wherefore? Because then when my limbs were cut away piece by piece, had I been bound by the distinctions aforesaid, feelings of anger and hatred would have been aroused in me. Subhuti, I remember that long ago, sometime during my past five-hundred mortal lives, I was an ascetic practicing patience. Even then was I free from those distinctions of separated selfhood.

Note: It is extremely difficult to find useful material on spirits, and Buddhism (and Hinduism) are few were there can be illustrated human – spirit interaction. Some Buddhist sutras are such, and it is wise to mention a note about this, to increase understanding and to be thankful for the little and hard to find information, and for me to make the obscure writings and story methods more digestible and useful. Sifting through so much useless information and history to find the few gems that can help sometimes to shed more light.

The different eyes humans can have

The different eyes humans can have. Excerpts from the Diamond Sutra:

"Let us look further into the five eyes. Are they produced from within or do they come from outside? The five eyes are not produced from within; nor do they come from outside: nor do they exist in the middle. Cultivate, use effort, and when your skill is sufficient you will have them naturally. Before sufficient skill is attained, no amount of seeking will cause them to function. Seeking is false thinking. Seeking without the thought of seeking brings a response.

In what way does one apply make an effort to open one's eyes?

You need to be wise in managing affairs, and wise in cultivation. It is wise to recognize what is good and then courageously and vigorously work toward it. The characteristic of wisdom is to recognize and vow to cut off and cast out what is bad. Realizing something is good and yet not acting in accord with it is the characteristic of stupidity. It is stupid to recognize that something is bad business and still go ahead and become involved in it. If you are stupid, it is not easy to obtain the five eyes. "In order to obtain them, everything you do must be done extremely clearly. You must be very precise and cannot be confused. What do the five eyes do?

The wisdom eye contemplates the nature of the Dharma realm. In so doing, the wisdom eye is complete with all aspects of wisdom.

When you wish to consult the Buddhist sutras, you must use a book. With the dharma eye, however, you do not need to read the sutras, because you can see the Buddha-dharma throughout all of empty space, everywhere throughout the Dharma realm. There are sutras everywhere. So it is said that the dharma eye completely illuminates the marks of all dharmas."

"The Buddha eye enables you to understand the true meaning of all Buddhadharma. Those of you who wish to attain the Buddha eye should remember that it is located between your eyebrows. Otherwise on the day when an eye appears in that place you will utterly panic and wonder, "How did I grow another eye?" My telling you in advance is to spare you any fear.

The dharma eye can thoroughly investigate everything. People's prior causes and subsequent results, the penetration of past lives, the penetration of the heavenly eye, all are completely understood. The Buddha eye is extremely wonderful and inconceivable. It can see things with form and things without form, with a power several million times greater than that of the flesh eye.

If you obtain the five eyes, you should protect them carefully. How should you protect them? By continuing to nourish your good roots. Cultivate blessings and wisdom. Those of you who have not obtained the eyes need to work hard and develop blessings and wisdom.

When your blessings and wisdom are sufficient your five eyes will open."

God and the Prophets

Why include a chapter or the subject of god and the prophets in a book on psychiatrical engineering? Historically and until now, as practiced in many countries and cultures, the issue of spirits is intimately linked to religion. And since the subject of this book is in great part about spirits, it is important to have some background into the subject, and also to serve as a warning and help focus the mind a little. It does not hurt to have this understanding and discussion. But also, it should not lead us away from our focus on psychiatry thru physics, that is, we can talk all we want about spirits and religion, but we want our search and focus to be purely through the path of physics as we outlined in our central thesis.

The first question

The first essential question to ask: who created you as a human? Is it random evolution that led to who and what you are right now? Or is it even possible to know answer to such query with certainty? On the question of certitude, would you find anyone to stand as a credible witness to authenticate such claims? Deduction, induction, interpolation, and myriad ways of logical thinking can take you so far. But, can you really know the truth without any shadow of a doubt?

The other part of the question is, if an intelligent being/s created you, then who created your creator? How did he/she/they come into existence? Extending the question further, who created the creator who created your own creator?

No matter what possible answer/s you might get, here's a scenario. When someone comes to you and says, "I created you," you may politely give this response, "If you created me, then may I ask who created you?" Further, you may say, "So you created me. Did you want to create a dumb robot or a smart one? A robot in your own image? If you wanted to create a smart robot just like you, then you should not be surprised if I am asking you these questions. But, if all you wanted was a worshipping robot who would serve as your slave, then you are talking to the wrong robot. So, you created something worthy of respect, and that is what I hope you can see and should expect here." And by the way, whoever created the creator, can create either one who is like him/her or one who is better than him/her.

Of course, on the other side, when part of the spirit world opened up to me, I saw the flip side of this. As far as I can tell, the high spirits, who made all their resources available to me, helped me in this hell I was suffering, but I cannot be sure. It is a hidden world, but one which is greatly intertwined with ours. And it is supposedly meant for the benefit of both human beings and the high spirits. Since I did not create life, and they know so much more about it, they seem highly credible. Of course, this could have also been a malicious spirit ritual, and I was their victim. However, since I am still in the midst of it, I will reserve my final judgment.

Meeting a more intelligent creator or even your possible creator, should not be such a self-annihilating experience that breaks down your spirit and self-respect. It is necessary that you respect yourself always. You must know that you are a great being – this is whether you have been created by an intentional act or the result of randomness.

When you understand and feel this deeply, then you can show appreciation to a creator for having created such a special being. A being who has self-worth equal and thinks of him/herself as equal to any being. A being who possesses awe and love for a real or imagined creator/s. As stated in the book of Genesis in the Old Testament of the Bible, "God created humankind in his own image, in the image of God he created them."

Whether you love poetry, fiction, nonfiction and other forms of artistic expressions, you may certain words, acts and creations that are so beautiful. With appreciation, you have to love and respect all of them.

Evolution can lead to the idea of a creator or creators. Alternatively, a creator can use evolution as a method for creation and use it as a mechanism. So both creation and evolution are plausible answers. But neither answer is completely certain about the origin of ALL life. So, after having considered various views, the appropriate answer to the first essential question is, "I do not know." From there, you can allow the discussion to move on to a different subject.

Life, as humans experience it, is a product of conscious creation. As my personal experience (and this has nothing to do with my belief) has shown me, life has been engineered through a conscious intentional creation. As for the entire universe I am not sure, and so I cannot say that the same is true it. Yet, just like a human being is a creator of complex machines, and later may become a creator of new life, he/she is a product of conscious creation, as was shown to me. However, it leads us again to the question, are the creators of humans a product of conscious creation or of random evolution? The answer I got was that they were also asking the same questions. I do not know how anyone can know for sure the very beginning of creation, because there is always the question of "who created the creator?" In addition, how could anyone have been there at the beginning of time to testify about it? Therefore, how does one know if there was a beginning or not? The only sure thing I know is that I do not know, and I don't know how anyone can know the answers. Interpolation, extrapolation and deduction cannot give certainty. Hence, the ultimate question of whether the whole of the universe (not restricted to some life forms only, such as humans and spirits) is a product of an intentional act or of a random one is not resolvable. Beyond that, I really don't know.

I do not know when the universe began, or if there was a beginning. It seems like there is plenty of time (all the time) in the world for anything to come into existence, intently or randomly. The universe may not even know about time, so these questions are unanswerable. If the universe had all the time, all events are possible to occur, no matter how seemingly complicated or strange these events are. Speaking of probability, if a random event is likely to occur every year and another event every one billion years, from one perspective, it may make no difference, since there is plenty of time for both events to occur. To say a year is shorter than a billion years can be immaterial. This is because, in either case, both events are equally likely that they will occur. The universe has billion, billion, billion, billion, billion, billion, (you get the point) of years in its past and future. Both events, no matter how likely or unlikely to occur, are equally likely that they will occur. The universe has all the time in the world in it! Or has it? Again, the appropriate answer is, "I do not know."

_____

Dangers in religions

Religions usually are meant to bring forth some useful values. Most importantly, they reveal important information about the spirit world which is inaccessible to most people. Yet, when you read carefully and analytically, you may find many conflicting facts and non-logical statements. Hence, it is wise to learn from the good parts and leave the rest behind. Maybe, out of a thousand pages, you may find only a few pages that are relevant. To illustrate this, read the following story from the Old Testament Bible – the basis of the "holiday of sacrifice" celebrated by Muslims yearly.

From:

http://www.rationalchristianity.net/abe_isaac.html

_____

Genesis 22:1-12

Sometime later God tested Abraham. He said to him, "Abraham!"

"Here I am," he replied.

Then God said, "Take your son, your only son, Isaac, whom you love, and go to the region of Moriah. Sacrifice him there as a burnt offering on one of the mountains I will tell you about."

Early the next morning Abraham got up and saddled his donkey. He took with him two of his servants and his son Isaac. When he had cut enough wood for the burnt offering, he set out for the place God had told him about. On the third day Abraham looked up and saw the place in the distance. He said to his servants, "Stay here with the donkey while I and the boy go over there. We will worship and then we will come back to you."

Abraham took the wood for the burnt offering and placed it on his son Isaac, and he himself carried the fire and the knife. As the two of them went on together, Isaac spoke up and said to his father Abraham, "Father?"

"Yes, my son?" Abraham replied.

"The fire and wood are here," Isaac said, "but where is the lamb for the burnt offering?"

Abraham answered, "God himself will provide the lamb for the burnt offering, my son." And the two of them went on together.

When they reached the place God had told him about, Abraham built an altar there and arranged the wood on it. He bound his son Isaac and laid him on the altar, on top of the wood. Then he reached out his hand and took the knife to slay his son. But the angel of the LORD called out to him from heaven, "Abraham! Abraham!"

"Here I am," he replied.

"Do not lay a hand on the boy," he said. "Do not do anything to him. Now I know that you fear God, because you have not withheld from me your son, your only son."

_____ end of quote

Now, reread this story with this in mind:

A father hears a voice telling him to kill his son as a sacrifice to the one who spoke. The father proceeds to prepare to kill his innocent son.

Regardless of who that voice was, god or otherwise, would a father kill his innocent son, and in a sinister way, for any reason at all?! Would you kill your son or daughter if anyone told you to do so for no reason other than sacrifice? Is this something that one should do? On top of all this, is this a good example of parent's behavior to promote and celebrate?

Yet that is what some religions and people love and celebrate.

Is anyone thinking? Are these people rational? Or are they blinded with fear by their religions?

Any wonder some religions, cultures, countries do not allow proselytization? Why should you hear any alternative information or view on a subject?

Dangerous beings they are, and they act based on their faith. So, you think all cultures, religions or teachings are equally deserving of the same consideration? Please be thoughtful and honest with yourself at least, let alone with others.

From what I know, the Jain religion insists that you think and use logic to guide you wherever the path leads.

The nature of god/gods

You do not know anything about god for sure – what he looks like, what he favors and dislikes, the nature of his life. In the following examples, we see an angry and violent god, as well as one who is incapable of interfering:

An angry god: he kicks Adam out of Garden of Eden for not respecting his request about eating the fruit of a specific tree (based on the Old Testament of the Bible).

A god who is incapable of interfering with the affairs of men: the devil tortures Job, and god cannot interfere. Or maybe he thinks it is all right to torture a human being as a test of devotion (based on the Old Testament of the Bible)

A god who urges to start a war: Krishna expounds the eternal dharma to his warrior of light, Arjuna, tells him that sometimes one must fight a war, and tries to help him. (Mahabharat Gita)

A god who gives advice on fighting strategy: he commands his people to blow the horns and the city walls will fall (Old Testament of the Bible)

Nature of the creator: I am the creator of all things and the destroyer of all things (Mahabharata Gita)

Be careful of talking about things of which are not knowledgeable.

God and War

In the Old Testament of the Jewish Bible, we find examples of God helping in wars. Likewise, in the Hindu religion texts, Bhagavad Gita, we find the god Krishna helping Arjuna and urging him to go to war, even though Arjuna does not want to fight his cousins. In Islam, the prophet Mohammed supposedly goes before a king and asks him to become a Muslim, otherwise the King will be attacked.

Jain and Buddhist views on gods

In general, Jainism and Buddhism supposedly minimize the role of god/gods. Regardless of contrary views, this can be a good thing. In what seems to be a formula in religions in terms of what you gain in knowledge, what you lose in reason and the connection to the heavens when you join a particular religion, the Jain religion seems to have it right in great part. Their attitude seems to be, in a nutshell: "we ask nothing of god, and we take care of ourselves. So we ask him to stay out of our business." Sad to say, there is a total lack of acknowledgement of life as a conscious creation, which should not diminish their logic. My experience clearly shows the reality of conscious creation, at least on the human level. But I digress.

About the afterlife

A human seems to have spirits who live with him – some came to him/her even before birth, at the time of his/her birth, or later on). Some spirits hold memory of your life just like a video recording, except that this recording system records all your senses (such as smell, touch, etc., that cannot be captured by the usual video recording system). This makes it possible to move all your memory, all its finest details and its continuity, from your body, specifically upon the time of your physical death. Your physical body is part of you, and when it is gone, you lose a major part of you, but it may not be important. It is like losing an arm and still thinking you have it (like what some people suffer when they lose a limb, which is called a phantom limb.) Similarly, if you want to, you can recreate the sensation of your body and its shape from complete memory. But the spirits I saw have very flexible and detached parts, so that it is almost meaningless to speak of a human body shape after death, as these spirits can almost assume any shape. This is what I saw through the pinhole I was looking through, but I could never be sure if it is true, or completely true. I tell you what I saw and experienced to the best of my knowledge, even though this information can be, at times, extremely incomplete. So the experience is as if your main spirit, which is a major part of you and which feels and sees along with you during life, lives in this other world. This other world can be the body of another human being (some call transmigration, or to a central location where there are systems for what happens to you and where you live after). There is a lot that I saw and experienced and this barely covers any of it. But I am not interested in writing more about this. My thinking is that when we develop the tools to find and communicate with these spirits directly, that is in very transparent way, and these spirits can relay all the information we ask about as needed. Dealing with spirits through any other way than in direct one and using modern equipment (as I have discussed in other parts of this book) can be very dangerous to the well-being of a human, since he/she will not be able to distinguish between good and evil spirits, as well as the many types of spirits. It is like talking on the phone where you cannot be sure who is on the other end and who they can imitate any sound and project any image or video into a human being's eyes. It is also easy to get sucked in into this world and lose focus of the outside world. I am absolutely against such an experience or experimentation, under any circumstance, except that which I state in the book. I hope my warning is clear enough!

Transmigration of spirits

Transmigration of spirits is that when a spirit moves from one being to another, while alive or typically upon death. In the west and much of the east, such knowledge is practically non-existent. In the Philippines, some families practice transmigration as part of their family tradition. So when a family member dies, another family member, an aunt or uncle maybe, is present in a ritual practice to welcome the dead person's spirit into their body. Some also talk to this spirit soon after to confirm the identity of the spirit. While the understanding of transmigration seems more common in Thailand, I was surprised to see it in the Philippines and practiced to such a level. Also surprising is the amount of cultural knowledge and acceptance of the existence of "the third eye" in the Philippines.

The spirit world can run in parallel to the human world

This is one of the strangest concepts I experienced about the spirit world – and a difficult one to explain. I do not know if this experience is universal or it only happened to me, although it seems to be the norm.

How do I explain this concept: that the spirit world runs in parallel to the human world? I will try several analogies first. Some computers have redundant processors to do the same task at the same time in parallel. If one processor fails, the other continues to finish the job. Some computers can store the data to two hard drives or locations at the same time, in order if one location is damaged or affected, the data is safe in the other location. Sometimes, a task is divided by a processor into many other subtasks, so that they can be performed in parallel by many processors or computers. Similarly, a group of people may all participate in a single event not just for efficiency, but also for social bonding, such as in building a public courtyard or joining the family in a large event. In such an event, both a father and 3-year-old son can be participating in an event at the same time, but the father who has more experience is playing the role of a watch-over and of a more able participant with the 3-year-old son not necessary being aware of this. So both can be pulling on a rope, but playing somewhat different roles. The role of the father is unnoticed and may not be understood by the 3-year-old son, and his true role as the guardian or watch-over is neither known nor understood by the child.

So here I present many different forms of event parallelism, each very different in function or purpose. If a machine is created in our world, the same machine, in its equivalent spirit form, is created also at the same time. So when I operate a machine, there are spirits also that operate the spirit form of the machine at the same time. So I am using a computer, and my spirit, a different being, is using the spirit of the same computer, which is a different machine! A machine that is a computer, made by the same manufacturers, yet is composed of and made for the spirit world. To try even more to explain this strange concept, I will add this analogy. Imagine a person speaking in English, while there are two people listening, one who understands German only and another who understands French only. If there is a human or computer translating simultaneously every English word to German and to French, then these two strangers can understand fully and instantly what is being said. This translation is done in parallel, and all three people can communicate without a problem, even though they do not know one another's language. So when you look at a computer and its English keyboard, the spirit sees a keyboard made of different materials and utilizes a different language. Both machines are the same machine, but operates in different levels at the same time (or operates in different languages at the same time, English language and spirit language). Moreover, one operates as a silicon computer while the other as spirit-made-material computer. The same computer serving your needs also serves the spirit's needs. Yet another analogy is like you looking at the computer processor with your bare eyes and seeing nothing but silicon metal and carvings, while the spirits look with MRI of the processor chip and see an entirely different picture that is completely incomprehensible to your eyes. Spirits do have MRI eyes, but they have their particular vision systems that may be completely different from and more inclusive than what we can see. So we both live in the same world and operate the same machines, but these machines serve us differently. In addition, we see these machines and their operations in varied ways. Some may see what we see and much more, we do not know, while others may see less, etc. The important thing to understand is that we both see another person, an animal or a car while walking on the street, but these same objects are seen completely differently and as having different functionalities. Nevertheless, they are seen at the same time and in complete parallelism. So while we might see a human, a dog or a car, spirits can see other spirits inside that human, dog or car, and they know many different things which you do not know about these objects. For example, dog you see appear like a spirit to the spirits who can see its internal components. Parallel to the man you can see, the human spirit sees the counterpart and knows more or less based on their world. The car that you see looks like a solid metal object, while to a spirit, it can have a completely different representation and additional functionality which you are not aware off.

I did not want to write about this subject, because it adds complications to the book and may distract the reader to take a different direction. I thought that in time, when we start a direct communication with spirits, they themselves can better explain these and other things. But then again, I thought the book may be incomplete without me just barely touching on the subject. And it is important to know how evil spirits or other spirits can interfere in all manners of life forms and machines. Our worlds are inclusive of each other and intertwined. And they seem omnipotent even when they are not. Just like the army in a civil government can have all the power to destroy and control everything if they decide to and can possess advanced technology, secrets and abilities, they are completely under the control of civilians and civil government. These worlds, and I repeat what one said to me, are made for both our benefits and coexistence. Do not waste your time with useless speculation and focus on what I am asking you to do. When these spirits are located and communication starts in a scientific and clear manner, then and only then will a whole new world open up and reveal itself at its own pace, comfort, and in the proper manner.

Spirits control of earth beings, in host or from a distance

A spirit can be mobile or immobile inside a human being and animals. Some are immobile in human beings, and they can control and greatly affect another human being or animals. For example, they can make a dog bark, or go to a specific location, or act in a specific way, such as try to spontaneously mate with another dog. This shows enormous control. Similarly, this can happen to a cat or rat or fly or mosquito. I saw this numerous times! And some of these spirits can go and host inside that being, for example, a dog, and they can use it like a robot. The functionality inside these animals and inside human beings seems to be very well known. These functions and their locations are transparent to many of the spirit types in the spirit world. To make a human sneeze, say something, look somewhere, feel some feeling, and organize complex events on time involving many humans, animals, etc. seem trivial tasks for these spirits. There are many types of spirits and groups, and some know or can do so much more than other spirits. Also, there is a huge variety and many hierarchies amongst some group types. This is an extremely important subject that I may expand on later.

Some spirits are far more advanced than other spirits

Spirits can have many shapes and forms, but I will mention one spirit that was communicating with me early in my experience. He told me this, "I am a creature spread in space and time, and you cannot understand this." I truly did not understand much of this initially. Years later, after seeing and experiencing more, I began to understand some things, even though many times I was not told about these things explicitly. So for example, when I noticed that almost all spirits can spread their body in space like a cloud over a small or great distance, the concept became understandable. For example, an electromagnetic wave from your phone or TV station can spread in space over very small or very large distances and spaces, thousands or millions or billions of kilometers in distance or in size. But instead of a simple electromagnetic sine wave, if we think of an extremely complex electromagnetic-non-solid-state made structure having a foot on earth, its hand on the moon, its head on Mars, then we can understand that a real being can be like that. These spirits are spread in time because of their size and are composed of almost fluid-like structures and parts that seemingly can be separated yet stay connected. Their connection being remote control-type or something else, I do not know, and I wanted to know! I did not want humans to be at the mercy of anyone after suffering much and meeting others who suffered from spirits. Not wanting to digress, of course, such beings may not have or not need a mouth, hands or feet. I simply use this analogy to help you understand. Some consume energy, and I speculate that as they travel in space, and if such beings have an energy mouth, so to speak, their mouth can be on the head or hand or foot or can dynamically change location! Trying to make analogies is helpful to make you understand, but it can be used to illustrate that spirits are also or can be completely different in structure and their survival requirements. However, most of the spirits relating to daily life on earth seem to be engineered in animal shape or functionality in their essence, while the more elevated spirits have different shapes, functions or connections to one another and to humans. These spirits who are animal-like in shape, function or primitiveness seemed to have caused me much of the suffering. Some have evil intentions and enjoy their act. While others are wild, and their evilness comes from their wild nature. You cannot say a lion is evil because he attacks other animals to eat and also may attack you. It is his nature. Some spirits are like that, and if the spirit immune system which humans have collapses, as did in my case, a human can become prey to all kinds of evil or wild spirits. Another warning! This world is not to experiment with or speculate about carelessly. I only ask engineers and scientists to approach this world and to open the doors properly with the right methods and tools. This is extremely a serious issue and requires the most reverence, knowing still it is full of wildness and evil. You would not just open the door to a wild zoo and walk in. Also, residing there may be spirits of your dead relatives and spirits from your relatives, as well as spirits that may have created life themselves, other beings and possibly humans! You may get much help and guidance unknowingly if you keep proper attitude and understanding. This is not looking at a petri dish of bacteria culture, but of small entities, some maybe far more intelligent than you. But some are the evil ones we want to kill or control. So how do you approach this world which is not supposed to be approachable or available? I contemplated on this much, and I think the time has come for the two worlds to connect.

A single very tiny cell created you

A single very tiny cell created you. This cell duplicated and differentiated. It was the source, and it seemingly stayed in control of the whole process. A hierarchy seems to exist, and affecting this cell may have an effect all the others. All the others provide feedback and functionality to it. There is a system for feeding all the cells – the blood vessels system. There are sensations systems, such as the nerves system. There are biochemical systems that work with endocrines. There are others that are hidden, such as the spirit system or so far unknown systems, a there are others that can be operationalized.

The most important things about religion

The most important things about religion:

The existence of the spirit unseen world. Religion speaks about an unseen world of spirits that exists. But as I have come to know, these teachings can, for the most part, be erroneous. Erroneous or not, such a world exists, as I talk about it from personal experience. The Buddha, in the Sutra, reveals much.

The function of religion as I see it. Religion is to serve men, and not the other way around. So when Christ broke the religious rules of the Sabbath by working to help a person, he demonstrated a higher value than religion. Men is more important than religion. So you will not misinterpret, Christ on the other end of the scale indicated that a tree needs to be sometimes trimmed of branches to grow stronger. So do not make of Christ as a mindless socialist. And he advised to not bury your money but put it to use.

In addition, freedom is highest. This refers to freedom of choice and freedom to be left alone. The New Testament says: if you are not welcomed in a particular place, kick the dust off your sandals and leave.

So religion should not be about mindless emotions, but about what value it adds to human life. Many religions seem to subtract value. But those that add value should be selectively looked at and made use of.

Additions to the book, unedited and not placed in best location Sept 20, 2018

Note : These editions were made shortly after first publishing the book. I wanted to add them even if unedited and unorganized and not placed in best location in the book. I thought they may be useful. Should I be able to, I may revisit this in the future and fix.

Must add: Many spirit seem to live inside human Aura. They stay there until death. Aura, is partly or fully electromagnetic standing field. If you take a tree leaf, and cut it, you can see the cut area is still visible under certain light frequencies. Observe it over time as it decays, and how this field changes moment by moment to learn about electromagnetic objects and robots. Do the same for human skin and nails. For robotic movement, look at schools of fish and birds. Separate but connected. Develop analogous forms in purely electromagnetic moving fields.

Learn to generate shapes and motion from sets of simultaneous math equations. Start with very simple examples and add complexity.

Must add: Currently computer chips and TV screens are made from matrices of millions for transistors, etc. Some have plasma, etc. Use these as starting points to generate electromagnetic fields. Make these elements programmable for producing electromagnetic fields. Also create three dimensional arrays, or simply stack several tv screens as starting point. Try to generate interesting electromagnetic fields that will move and do special functions. Eventually, you will learn to create ones that will fly from the screen as a living robot. Use random generation and exploration. Surround the room by electromagnetic field detection to know when the computer has generated something interesting and can move in space controllably, etc...

Must add: to my credential. Programmed much of the "CRC Standard Mathematical Tables and Formulae", used as a reference by scientists. Incidentally, the head of math department in my university compiled the book. There, I studied mathematics for few years, and did the project completely on my own without help or knowledge of others, using the LISP computer language. A computer symbolic language used initially in the studies of artificial intelligence. Amusingly as a child, maybe 15 years old, I sold Hewlett Packard primitive calculators that unusually used Reverse Logic Notation, which my father brought from the USA. Later as an adult, learning a little bit of Thai language, I found out they use similar grammatical logic.

Must add: Spirits are extremely abundant, and are part of our invisible world. When a spirit moves from being to another, while both beings are alive, it is called transmigration, when they move to another being after death, and into a new born or in the womb, it is called reincarnation. Though one spirit from a being can have no, some, or most of that being's characteristics, so that when they move to another being, depending on this spirits strength, it can effect the new host little or greatly. When it effects them greatly, it can also give them the characteristics of the original being, and in some cases can share with them , the memory, so that the new being will gain knowledge about this other life, or past life. No moment in life can be duplicated completely, because doing so means, duplicating the entire universe as is for that moment. Bacteria in your body, neutrinos passing through your body, etc. Does your memory bank have this information and preserve it and it's physics effect on you. And when you die, your body dies and changes. A spirit can preserve in its memory or structure much of the physical and mental body, but It cannot duplicate it completely. So when transmigration or reincarnation happens, it is with those limits in mind.

Must add: Some old cultures had some good understanding that been lost with time: the culture of the Jain, in India, had the habit of nudity, especially for monks. The Hindu religion put images of men with erected penises on the walls of their temples, and taught about how to practice some sex positions etc. Neither nudity nor sex were subjects to shy about, but the opposite. Modern day Hindus to me seem so far removed and regressed from their old roots, they think and act like barbarians. Same for the old Greeks, compared to the modern day Greeks. And so is their knowledge of the celestial world. Today, people have much more advanced technology and because of that more wealth, and use this crutch as a substitute and alternate to good culture. With good culture you have more wealth, mental, physical and economic. Modern wealth is a great drug/opium, that mask the ills of modern society, and they are blinded by small successes from bigger successes. If you had no money and in need, and someone showed you a system and you made from it 100 money units, you may become very happy, so happy that you will sing the praises of this system, and will not consider anything else, even though there may be another system that will give you 1000 money units return, or eliminates need for much money, but demands more mental ability to understand. Little success deceives and becomes a wall to seeing much bigger success.

Must add: Even though my mental and real vision into this world and the celestial world maybe 1000 times greater than a normal human being, I am still looking through a pinhole into the celestial world, the spirit world, and my vision may be one million times less than theirs.

Must add: it is extremely important to understand the word "avatar". A being in heaven can be somewhat an avatar to a being on earth, or a being on earth can be somewhat of an avatar or like an avatar for a being in the spirit world, or both, that is, both beings, on earth and heaven, can be like avatars to each other. It can be much more complicated and different, but this minimal level of understanding is absolutely essential to an understanding to some of the things I talk about. More important to understand your importance as a being, and that you can be in charge when you understand. You can control instead of being controlled, or attempt to do that. Just because you are a child without understanding, it does not mean you are not protected by parents, and just because you are parents, it does not mean your understanding is complete, or that the armies rule even when they have the physical powers and state secrets. In a civil system, civilians rule. Do not be in fear of all this power or knowledge or hidden knowledge, all of this exists maybe to serve you. But this freedom you have and now are gaining greater understanding of, means also you are responsible for your own self, to strive to succeed on your own. Some want a formula for intervention between humans and avatars, or none, to preserve the separation wall and freedom. Others want different equations. Now you have a little sense of what is involved. Strive to make your part on earth, and let others do their part in the heavens. In my life, I sometimes had to read a book twenty times or much more, and every time I understood things I did not understand or see before. If you see something or a book that seems important, then it is worth spending the time on it, for understanding or enjoyment.

Must add: Extremely important. Why do people not see that some religions are useless for asking for help and miracles? Have they not tried enough to ask, or seen others ask without getting any immediate result? In Islam, I think it says Allah is capable of anything. In Christianity, Jesus says, whatever you ask in my name you shall receive. How many failures before they realize that there is something wrong with all this? Are these lies or misinformation? There is a separation wall in general between the spirit world and earth, and this wall is to preserve our freedom from intervention by spirits. The flip side of this is that spirits are not allowed to intervene in our world. Spirits told me the control between heaven and Earth does not allow this, to prevent anyone, no matter, from interfering in people's affairs, one way or the other. You have freedom, and this means you are responsible for yourself". Religion is one very minor component of earth heaven systems. A much bigger component is parents' spirits in heaven relation to children. Also the dead and dead family members system, etc. Also, and I could not assess completely, is protection of humans from the spirit world system. It is a form of security system. There is more, but is important to know, the importance of religion in these systems. This means that prayers etc., should be useless, especially if we care about our freedom. But the wall is broken sometimes by individual spirits or groups of spirits, for good or bad reasons. Just like you are bound by systems on earth, so are spirits. This is extremely important information to understand and remember. If you pray for help out of desperation, it is okay, and you may get results. But pray merely to connect to that other world, the world of loved ones and ancestors and good, and for being in awe of creation.

Must add: Random thoughts: I heard that these spirits which can morph into cloud like shapes and flexibilities are related to plasma in design. Exploring design using plasma may be useful in these regards.

Must add: Some of these spirits can use direct electric energy sources, such as phone battery, electric power lines, or running car engines.

Must add: Random thoughts: I changed my diets over the years based on best information I had. The last few years, my diet was like a vegan diet, then the last year's added animal products of milk and eggs of necessity I felt for protein when I did not find or could afford vegetarian substitutes. I switched to the last diets for two reasons: being told by spirits that meat eating spirits in heavens, by their nature, introduce the meat eating system into the body, which is a system of killing. To get fresh meat in general, you have to kill. The second reason was consideration of the question as to whether some animals have any feelings, especially empathy feelings. That is, put two chicken next to each other both eating, and kill one of them, will the remaining chicken react? If not, then maybe they do not have the important feelings I care about. So when people asked me if I was a vegetarian, I say I eat like one, but I am not, because in my thoughts I will eat meat if I have to, since I could not resolve these questions completely, but more importantly, I will more readily eat wild animals meat, carnivores, because that is these animals system. I will be treating these animals according to their system. Farm animals, bred for eating and without empathy feelings, are okay to eat if more healthy options are not available or if they are the best option.

Must add if already not included: Random thoughts: uneducated or improperly educated beings can be a great threat to your physical, mental, financial, economic, spiritual wellbeing, and freedom.

Must add for me and my children to know: Random thought: Blocking pain: I cannot think of the amount of harm and torture these spirits have done to me. To my body, and to my mind, and to my children. I cannot look, or don't want to look at this damage or try to remember for too long. It is very difficult.

Must add: How can you respect yourself if your body is not in good shape? Do you not need to question the amount of intelligence or education you have? When you look at another person in a very analytical way, and you see them out of shape, should this not cause a question about their education, intelligence or values? This is a most fundamental issue relating to human wellbeing and affairs. I would think your body and mind are extremely important. And if so, why are you not following priorities? And what does this tell me about you or your intelligence or your behavior or your values? The answer is that you are missing important qualities as a human, either in intelligence or values, or suffer events beyond your control that requires explanation.

Must add: To my biography section: As I try to recollect how my episode and the encounter with the spirit world started, and this is before I had any such knowledge or belief whatsoever of this world, and as I tried to make sense of it, it was a friend of mine that visited my house and started to work with me daily in my home office, and this lasted for a short period. Every day he worked in the adjacent office in my basement, and may eat with me and my wife in the house. I do not remember the exact stretch of time until I started experiencing strange things and events in my personal physical body and surrounding that eventually led to the spirit world opening before my eyes. This friend was not religious according to him even though he had a Jewish father and was of the

Jewish religion. As things began to unfold at the very beginning, in what seemed like a hallucinatic state, not necessarily a good one but the opposite, a voice came to me and at the same time drew the Star of David on my forehead, saying that "You are the chosen one". As I suffered during these months and years to follow with my condition, I do not remember the exact stretch of time after, that spirits, of living evangelical friends I had, came to me in a very strong presence doing many things that I did not understand the purpose of. These very close friends, that we have shared living quarters and time before, would among other things ask me to read from the New Testament bible citations or paragraphs. Some of it seemed as if I was being prepared to play the role of Jesus, or something to that effect. I did not understand what was going on and later on to start thinking if this was done in gest or as very good friends coming to rescue me from evil spirit that has come to me, or that these spirits had their own future designs for something to happen, or a combination of these possibilities. That is to say, something evil may have happened to me by an evil spirit coming to me as an individual act of that spirit or as part of a ritual, and then these spirits of friends and others coming to my rescue from this evil spirit or ritual. And I often wondered if these friendly spirits became part of the ritual knowingly, or unknowingly being misled to become part of this spirit world ritual. Sometimes the damage is done with the first hit and it is irreversible and too late for repair, and the only remaining option is to go along with the ritual, or rather than rescue the victim from the clutch of a wild evil spirit as you would from the clutches of a human caught by a lion and being chewed on, it is sometimes better to shoot that person in the clutches of the lion and the lion itself if you know you cannot save that person properly, with him coming out from this event without hands or feet and so badly damaged and mangled. I still until now do not know the answer even though I felt that many spirits that talked to me knew the complete answer but would never tell me even though I wanted to know and I asked. Many times I felt very strongly that I was being an unwilling part of a ritual in the spirit world. Sometimes a social ritual can be for choosing a man or a woman to be sacrifice for the gods, or sometime the ritual can be for choosing a person who will be the president of the village. I did not want to be part of either ritual and felt I was fighting the ritual itself. I did not want to be the sacrifice for a god, or the president of the village so to speak. As an unwilling participant being drafted into this I was fighting the existence of the ritual itself. Also, sometimes I felt like the devil came to me and showed me the spirit world and its kingdoms and saying it's all yours just come along and accept the system and what's happening to you. And at times I heard what I thought was my own holy spirit that protects me telling me that "I am showing you the world, all of it as I tried to help you get out of the fall and the evil that has come to you and as I tried to free you from this evil that has come into your body, and sense it will take a long time in the fight to do it I wanted you to know exactly your situation and see this other world so you can understand what has happened to you and what is happening to you and the struggle to save you.

Must add: Think and be careful: The Vatican imprisoned the famous scientist Galileo in the 17th century AD for saying the earth revolves around the sun. The church taught that the sun revolve around the earth which was later proven to be false. Think. Be careful of what you hear and what you read. If the church meant that the earth was the center of the spirit world, that is a completely different issue. But this takes the subject far out of any normal human experience and is irrelevant to what I am trying to warn about. One more time, think, question, be careful, to hopefully have some understanding.

Must add: I was told that communication between spirits is at ultra-high frequency. At the molecular vibration level. Another spirit said to look in the ultrasound spectrum for spirit – human unwanted chatter.

Must add: Random thought: Sometimes, creating an intelligent machine necessitates that it's all its components have the same intelligence. Even creating a machine for the simplest of tasks, can require this kind of design. The smallest component is as intelligent as any of the others. At that point, the machine may take on different characteristics. One example is biological beings where the smallest component is the cell where all the cells have equal intelligence but differentiate to specialize on single and simple tasks.

Must add: In the section about remote vision and cell phone technology of seeing all people in a building say: remote vision, and communication are present in human, in the spirit subconscious part. Just like nowadays cell phone have such remote vision a communication and you in turn have these abilities because you own a cellphone, same with your innate or spirits that come to you, they provide you with similar and other capabilities. And though these abilities are in you, many over time can atrophy or intentionally be deprecated over time. Atrophy because of lack of use, just as I turn off the "locate nearby friends service" application in the cell phone to maintain privacy. I do not want my friends and others to know my every move and location. So you can see why many people do not use this very advanced form of remote vision even though it is readily accessible in the unconscious part of our being. You want to see me remotely and without my permission? You can, but I do not like this, and I will turn off this feature in my body or create counter measures to maintain privacy or even security. Or human features can be deprecated because the powers that be in the spirit world may have interests in this happening. There are systems and controls in the spirit world, much as you should expect any beings to have. And it is connected with our system, the unseen one. I personally experienced these things, intensively, but better left for future days and others to reveal completely, as soon as we establish "formal" and "credible" communication with that world, which I hope will be soon. You can ask or discover and they will reveal and answer. The problem is a technical one. Their works is super tiny, where universes for them can fit on the head of a pin. And how do you know which is talking to you, when they do? These problems are solvable to a great degree. We can try, and they should also.

Must add: Jesus in the story of the servant who after the master left the house in the hands, of the servants, the servants took over the house as their own. In the spirit world, there are things very difficult to explain, but I put these for the record and for my children to know. An army in a civil country, though possessor of great power, control, equipment and secrets, can be subject to the control of a single civilian man who has no comparable physical power or resources. But they obey him. A child in a family may be given by the father and mother all the attention and resources, and their life if needed, even though the child has no power and no awareness of all this. So do not be surprised to know that you as a human, have incredible powers protecting you and resources under your control, that you are completely unaware off. And if someone comes to take over these hidden treasures that belong to you, as the servants in that house tried to take over, do not forget that the House is yours and was given to you by your family, or unknown family. And further if they said to you "you are a god" and can rule the world completely as wish, you can reply when you become educated: and how can I rule over others as I wish? Am I not subject to understanding, that if I am smart enough to rule, I am smart enough to know that I should not rule over another man? Because I would not want a god or a man to rule over me. If a good constitution has rules that begin with these words "the government shall not", "shall not interfere", "shall not do this or that", rules that show that rules should be imposed on government not people, then this is a good start of understanding. And by the same logic, how can a god rule over man. A god can see that ruling over man is a bad idea. And if so, if I were a ruler or a commoner, the result should be same. That is, how a wise ruler would act and therefore, why making me a god, other than to burden me with responsibility too great, equal to that power. Do you understand all these things combined together in one idea? And when the spirits in the spirit world think they own you, I think they should know better.

Must add: the Quran has many chapters named as "The image (photo) of the cow", "The image (photo) of the Ant" etc. For Muslims holly words, for whatever reason, put under the title of animals. The Bible of the Christians, The New Testament, has its most chapters named as "John", "Mathew", etc. The world of animals is that of power, and authority, and the world of humans, should be about freedom and intelligence. In the Jewish old testament Bible, Moses raised a snake, to fight snakes, but Jesus said to paraphrase: we should raise a human instead, as Moses raised a snake. As human, we have choices as to who we raise. And why we choose one and not the other. It is my understanding that Buddhist lower the importance of gods, and Jain religion sees even lesser need for gods if at all. They make distinctions between an absolute god and the world full of spirits. My experience shows me that life is a creation and even as a creator one may create and does not govern the creation, but lets the creation govern itself.

Must add: in the Jewish old testament Bible, there are several mentions of The Lord being defeated because the enemy had chariots made of iron. Reference: Old Testament: Book of Judges 1:19 "The Lord was with the men of Judah. They took possession of the hill country, but they were unable to drive the people from the plains, because they had chariots fitted with iron." (https://biblehub.com/niv/judges/1.htm). Conclusions: 1. Their Lord fights. 2: Iron made a difference between winning and losing.

Important to note: Many third eye cultural and religious information seems to have been intentionally atrophied. Hindu third eye painted on the forehead between the eyes of their people without knowledge of what the symbol is. Buddhists third eye on Buddha statues, Jewish blocks worn on third eye forehead location, etc.... Who is doing this? Why? Why do they want to hide this intrinsic function and knowledge? Is it meant to be hidden? Is it not part of the design?

Must add: when some spirits come into a human body, such as the spirit of a dead relative, it comes with the understanding of obeying a specific system to be allowed in. One of these requirements is to observe silence. They have access to hearing and seeing, and can live like watching a movie all the time, the life of a human. But with a schizophrenic person or a voice hearer, the system is broken. But this presents an excellent opportunity for scientists to listen to spirits because some stop observing silence. Use this fantastic opportunity to find some of these spirits!

Must add: Spirits seem to have different types of vision systems. Some spirits seem to have spirits matching the human visual system where only certain light frequencies are seen, while others have very different vision, like x-ray, MRI, ultrasound, etc. Human can add these vision ranges using equipment, now bulky, but they can. However, many spirits, seem to see with eyes only but with their whole body. They form like a cloud body that can wrap around an object, just like ultrasound waves, to see the whole object. Just like we can see with our entire body an object when we touch it, such as closing our eyes and feeling it with our hands to know (shape and texture), they can know with their whole body, shape, texture, color, etc. It is like the whole body is composed of eye vision cells so-to-speak, but much more! So an ultrasound wave can see a room and wrap itself around objects and go thru objects to see the inside, in case of some spirits, the wave is the spirit. Spirits seemed to have wave-like-body in function. And of course, human analogy is used to make you understand, because their body may have no cell structure at all. A single wave when touched in any of its body, can feel the location of touching, etc. Again, only analogies are being used to help avoid boxing your thinking as relating to form and function, material and construction

Very important: most effective massages by far were when I had three or four people together giving me the massage. They surrounded me. One per foot or hand, head, etc. It was incredible the results. It is like having four bodyguards around you, surrounding you physically and being able to touch you without inhibition, while surrounding the enemy evil spirits. Very dramatic results. The sad part is that I could only afford this for a brief period of time. But it is the best money spent by me. I do not know how many sufferers can afford this, if it was found to be useful for them.

Must add: In the body, some spirits live in a still form, that is their preferred state, which can be sticky fluid like. From this, they can transform to other forms. In fluid form, it looked like sometimes, many of them can be together, so that they may look like a drop of fluid but is composed of millions of spirits, or only one, that can move as fluid or become airborne. An analogy is that water is fluid but when very hot it becomes airborne vapor. But these I think are of material with different properties. Other spirits have more specific forms and prefer to be in motion. Both types have unusual properties I could not explain and was not explained to me, in how they can become like a cloud, change shape, separate body parts, yet somehow keep integrity as one body. I only once saw in a scientific documentary an animal or insect that was like Mercury metal fluid element. As soon as it separated from the main body, it had a form onto itself, and could join back into the main body acting as one body. I could not find years later what this specie was when I wanted to find out the name to add to the book. By the way, some of these spirits have access to incredible databases or ways to find almost anything by broadcasting, etc.. Example: if they need a person, with blond hair, nose that curves down, green eyes, short, looks like a specific individual, etc. They can find it. They can arrange for events to occur at certain times, by affecting people, animals, and other things animate or seemingly inanimate objects as well. And they also change from liquid to gas like forms with shapes. So looking at a liquid in the spine or brain or inside a cell, you maybe looking at them and not know that these are new life forms. How to coax them to move, or react, or change form is not something I know. Similarly looking at electromagnetic structures. Most important and odd is that while you may be looking at them and not know what you are looking at, they may be looking back at you and know what they are looking at. One thing to note is that under normal circumstance, when spirits entering the body through the legal route, they are to observe silence and local rules. Which makes it difficult to deal with in your search. However, in cases of schizophrenia, the rules maybe broken by some, which can be a rare opportunity. When we are at this stage of inquiry, at such a level of life forms and how they relate to us, a great deal of respect is required. That is just how it is!

Extremely important to understand: you should by now know there are two systems, to simplify, we call earth and spirits systems. They are intimately connected, for the most part. When you have a system that is connected to you, and you are unaware of and cannot control, that can be very dangerous or threatening. As such, you should also know, there is a security system to control and manage the spirit world. Just as on earth, it is a security system by necessity, and protects us. Just as children are protected by parents and can be completely unaware of the world and how it functions. Adults are protected by and from the spirit world and are completely unaware of how it functions. The disagreement can be as on earth, for how the security system should be. A dictatorship of sorts, a more accommodating democracy with freedom but has cost of security dangers, or other very complicated systems unknown to us. We need protection from evil spirits. We need some system or mechanism for this.

It can be enough for you to know this. Just like having police or an army. If they are very good at their job, they will not interfere in your life or even noticed, while they do their job of keeping you safe from evil and offending doers (spirits). When the system breaks down or have individual failure, it can be schizophrenia or it can be more subtle and unnoticeable, and thus very damaging at large. If the break is intentional and ritualistic, it can be a disaster for the individual, as seems to be the case for me, and a revelation for humanity. The spirits in my case seems to have taken a horrible ritual event by evil, or an evil devastating act, or acts by uneducated well-meaning spirits, and turned this lemon into somewhat of a lemonade; as a caring act, and used it to inform humans of the other world, and their very intimate connection to it. This can happen every few thousand years, or every kalpa maybe. So security is very important, and this is not an intellectual toy or subject to take lightly, as I have warned most firmly. When you pray, even falsely, you are still showing reverence and acknowledge meant to this other world, whether you do it knowingly or unknowingly. Some form of this seems needed just to remember this fact: another unseen world is part of us, intimately, and can be full of love and can be full of evil.

must add: extremely important: Unless we see these spirits under a microscope, so to speak, and they possibly also help in this, then our relations with religion and its spirit world is that of a master - robot, or master-slave or as an improper parent-child. But under the microscope, we look at them, and they look at us, and we know it is a system for both of us, based on respect, love, and kinship. If it is not, I will fight them, and I hope good spirits who agree with this view help. This is to me the central issue of the mystery of life and creation.

Kalpa, is one of the most beautiful words I have come across. If some beings live few years, and we as humans few more or a hundred, what can you say about creatures that have life cycles and live for billions of years? or more? If you are intelligent, how possibly intelligent are some of these creatures? A billion, trillion times more? The word Kalpa can begin to mean what is possible.. and with that much time at hand, all is possible. And some of these beings are strongly connected to us. I want or expect the relationship to be based on respect. They may know so much more and be so much stronger, but I expect they will want the same relation with other beings that may still be smarter and stronger than them. There is a cutoff point at which you realize that relations between intelligent beings should be based on respect, not power. Love, kinship, are a bonus.

Must add to the book: if you want to pray, it is for being in awe of creation, and out of love, Add " life in my experience seemed like a flower closed, and there comes a time when it opens up, and after, it looks at itself, its inside, and sees it, and sees itself and its secrets and understands, as if seeing inside it a label inscription saying 'made by God/Gods'". And with me, spirits who know about these issues and affairs of life, not only visited or spoke to me, but showed me. I said before, and re-emphasize, even when this is the case, you should ask other questions. Such as "Who made this god/gods/creatures/beings?" This is important. If a father's sperm and a mother's egg created you, and a mother brought you to this world, you lose neither love nor respect for knowing this, but have more of it, love, respect, and in this case also have awe.

Must add: With you or without you, life goes on. And whatever generated you, can do it again, or do it better. Given enough time, all things seem possible. Do not show yourself greater than me, the universe that led to you may do it again or do it better.

Must add to the book: a single cell created you and maybe in control of the other cells derived from it, cell differentiation, vision, hearing, sensations, etc. If you can access the proper part of a cell or this specific original cell, you may have access or controller to all this, or most, or essential functions. Touching or sending a message to the proper part of the cell may do this. Messenger protein agents are now known. Electromagnetic communication is not. It should be investigated. And a structure in space or in the body near the cell, seems to be used as a nesting area for spirits and karma related activities. Investigate locations, extremely tiny, and sever or block these connections to block the nesting of these beings. Destroy if you can. Strengthen your own natural faculties not their avatar faculties and functions. Those meddling middleman spirits sent to you from birth or before, to eventually take over completely. Reject them in to your sayings. Do not accept things you do not know or understand.

Must reiterate: Sakyamuni Buddha was tortured by Mara and his daughters says the LalitaVistara Sutra. At times, his body was so frail and maybe not thinking well that spirits had to advise him what to eat to restore his health. He was fighting in the spirit world. He expressed his fight and will in the beautiful words of the Sutra saying "it is possible they can catch the wind with a lasso, or draw words in the sky ….. but you, and countless beings like you can never move me from under this tree." And when he was done meditating, he had to put up with people showing lack of respect. He had to defend who he is and credentials to Deer Park athetics, and tell others how to address him properly and respectfully. As for Jesus, little was not said or done to him in lack of respect and to cause fear and later in torture. You know how I feel about those spirits and their world? I want to destroy them. They tried to harass me and rape me in public, and while using the toilet, and while eating, talking or having sex. It is evil you cannot imagine. I hope you will act on my advise and begin the search for them. So that no one else have to go through this again, and suffer from these evil bastard beings. When you pray to those in the spirit world, pray that they will help make this world visible to scientists. So that humans are not held hostage and vulnerable to those beings, and to take away their simple advantage of being invisible. It is like searching for a bacteria or a virus or a radio signal. You may look a very long time at frequency ranges, and wave shapes, and times the signal is used, but with guidance or even straight information, the search can end quickly. Demand!!! These being that enter and interfere in our bodies become known!!!!

Must add: it has been my experience, that those spirits sent to you at birth or before, from the heavens , as seemingly a mandatory process, that continually connect a human to the spirit world. However, this initial spirit, which some label as their "personal god" or "Holly spirit" or "shadow" or maybe "personal manager of heavenly affairs", is meant only for you, as a special function being. However, these beings have rules and regulations, and behaviors encoded in them, and these behaviors I disagreed very strongly with. Behavior that is partly from the animal world unfit to be combined with human values, such as animal body language. The are controlled manufactured beings and I have caught that they be replaced by more appropriate version. Better yet maybe, if they do not send any of them at all, but I do not know enough on the subject to be this categorical.

Must add, and is repetitious: it is great idea, to destroy your karma, and better to not give it a place to nest and grow. It is animal like automata. Humans are better off without it. We should not be inflexible and bound by anything rigid, let alone bad and rigid. Or be controlled by things they do not know first-hand or understand.

Must add: a person can look at an object, an image of the object, or the memory of the object. The idea of mapping is extremely important to expand a person's mental ability. Looking at a pipe, or its photo on a computer screen, or at its memory inside the silicon chip, are completely different things, but they are connected. Mapping one shape to another, one idea to another, one map to another, one logic maybe to another, etc. It is important to have a grasp of mentally and if possible mathematically.

Many spirits that come to a human seem to reside in the Aura of the human. I experienced others that came to the ears and could speak directly, and others in the base of the sexual area at the chakra there. In my case, I think the transmission of sound or sensation was not a microwave wave energy or such, but some of these electromagnetic beings physically touched the correct cell and correct part of the cell in the ear to transmit or generate the voices or sensations.

More additions: December 2018

A traditional faith healer can sometimes be well connected to the spirit world. Spirits in him can see the spirits in you and see the problem internally in you, and his spirits will fix the problem. No magic in this. Few faith healers maybe this effective. I knew several people who experienced spirit problems or knew someone very close to them with a problem and was healed this way. Again, this is not magic or mystery, I just told you the mechanism of what happens when they are successful or can solve these types of problems. My experience and spirits told me this. Incidentally, there are locations that get corrupted, damaged, or emptied, in parts of the human body, in the most delicate control area of the body, that spirits know about, and where some types of spirits are needed there or the opposite (should not be there). These traditional healers with their seeing spirits spot the problem and may provide the solution. Although this is a mechanical process, in that world, and can work, it cannot be called science until the process is completely observable and repeatable in laboratory. I hope in the near future, it will be so.

Must add: Philippines seems like a very good place for the center to be located. The people here seem be greatly aware of The Third Eye. Culturally, they are aware of spirits and their interactions. Unlike other countries such as Thailand, which has great awareness of spirits, the Pilipino in my limited experience seem to be willing to act on their knowledge, maybe because they are Christians, which may have different effect on them than the practice of Buddhism. They generally speak English. Respectful of the spirit world. The only weakness I see is technological, in terms of advanced equipment, technology, and financial capabilities. These can be remedied by cooperation with other places and help. It is important to have the surrounding culture of engineers and scientists be accepting seriously to look into the subject. In these countries, it should be easy, as opposed to western countries.

Conclusion: The most important personal statement I can make from my experience is that these spirits are real. I interacted with them in nearly every way. Just as I interact with normal beings. It may be a most unusual experience for a human, but it is real. I do not know how to stress this enough or elaborate on it. I do not know how often the spirit world opened up in this manner in the past or to this extent, in a period of one hundred or thousand or ten thousand years or much more, and if it is a singular or nearly singular event, in any way, it did happen!!! The results may be quite dramatic for the future. I do not know. I am tired, and leave the rest for you to discover or deal with. I am exhausted and nearly completely destroyed from the experience.

Historic notes

Discovery of Bacteria:

https://explorable.com/discovery-of-bacteria says:
"Antony Leeuwenhoek was the first person to see bacteria. Through the late 1670s, he sent comprehensive data and detailed drawings of his sightings of bacteria and algae to the Royal Society in London. Throughout his lifetime Leeuwenhoek remained devoted to the scientific research and made several vital discoveries."

It adds "Van Leeuwenhoek discovered "protozoa" - the single-celled organisms and he called them "animalcules". He also improved the microscope and laid foundation for microbiology. He is often cited as the first microbiologist to study muscle fibers, bacteria, spermatozoa and blood flow in capillaries. Although, he did not have much education or a scientific background, yet he defied all odds to be reckoned as a great scientist through his skillful observations, insight and unmatched curiosity."

Discovery of Virus:

https://en.wikipedia.org/wiki/History_of_virology
It says "Despite his other successes, Louis Pasteur (1822–1895) was unable to find a causative agent for rabies and speculated about a pathogen too small to be detected using a microscope.[1] In 1884, the French microbiologist Charles Chamberland (1851–1931) invented a filter – known today as the Chamberland filter – that had pores smaller than bacteria. Thus, he could pass a solution containing bacteria through the filter and completely remove them from the solution.
In 1876, Adolf Mayer, who directed the Agricultural Experimental Station in Wageningen was the first to show that what he called "Tobacco Mosaic Disease" was infectious, he thought that it was caused by either a toxin or a very small bacterium. Later, in 1892, the Russian biologist Dmitry Ivanovsky (1864–1920) used a Chamberland filter to study what is now known as the tobacco mosaic virus. His experiments showed that crushed leaf extracts from infected tobacco plants remain infectious after filtration. Ivanovsky suggested the infection might be caused by a toxin produced by bacteria, but did not pursue the idea.[3]
In 1898, the Dutch microbiologist Martinus Beijerinck (1851–1931), a microbiology teacher at the Agricultural School in Wageningen repeated experiments by Adolf Mayer and became convinced that filtrate contained a new form of infectious agent.[4] He observed that the agent multiplied only in cells that were dividing and he called it a contagium vivum fluidum (soluble living germ) and re-introduced the word virus. Beijerinck maintained that viruses were liquid in nature, a theory later discredited by the American biochemist and virologist Wendell Meredith Stanley (1904–1971), who proved

that they were in fact, particles.[3] In the same year Friedrich Loeffler (1852–1915) and Paul Frosch (1860–1928) passed the first animal virus through a similar filter and discovered the cause of foot-and-mouth disease.[5]

In 1881, Carlos Finlay (1833–1915), a Cuban physician, first conducted and published research that indicated that mosquitoes were carrying the cause of yellow fever,[6] a theory proved in 1900 by commission headed by Walter Reed (1851–1902). During 1901 and 1902, William Crawford Gorgas (1854–1920) organised the destruction of the mosquitoes' breeding habitats in Cuba, which dramatically reduced the prevalence of the disease.[7] Gorgas later organised the elimination of the mosquitoes from Panama, which allowed the Panama Canal to be opened in 1914.[8] The virus was finally isolated by Max Theiler (1899–1972) in 1932 who went on to develop a successful vaccine."

Cause of some ulcers:

A personal favorite and amusing story is when a relative of mine had ulcer and I had just read of research that it was actually a bacteria that causes it and not stress and advised taking antibiotics. Later, this is what happened according to this report by the Guardian newspaper https://www.theguardian.com/education/2005/oct/03/research.highereducation:
"Robin Warren, a pathologist from Perth, and Barry Marshall, a senior research fellow at the University of Western Australia, share the prize for their 1982 discovery of a bacterium, helicobacter pylori, which causes stomach inflammations and ulcers.
Prior to this discovery, it was generally believed that stress and lifestyle were the chief causes of stomach infections.
The Nobel assembly said the pair had used "tenacity" to challenge prevailing theories about stomach disease, making an "irrefutable case" that this bacterium caused more than 90% of duodenal ulcers and up to 80% of gastric ulcers. The discovery also challenged the prevailing treatments for ulcers. The committee said their pioneering discovery meant stomach ulcers were no longer a chronic, disabling condition, but a disease that could be cured."

Inquisition of Galileo:

From https://en.wikipedia.org/wiki/Galileo_affair and
https://en.wikipedia.org/wiki/Heliocentrism
In 1610, Galileo published his Sidereus Nuncius (Starry Messenger), describing the surprising observations that he had made with the new telescope, namely the phases of Venus and the Galilean moons of Jupiter. With these observations he promoted the heliocentric theory of Nicolaus Copernicus (published in De revolutionibus orbium coelestium in 1543). Galileo's initial discoveries were met with opposition within the Catholic Church, and in 1616 the Inquisition declared heliocentrism to be formally heretical. Heliocentric books were banned and Galileo was ordered to refrain from holding, teaching or defending heliocentric ideas (the astronomical model in which the Earth and planets revolve around the Sun at the center of the Solar System. Historically, heliocentrism was opposed to geocentrism, which placed the Earth at the center.)